YOGA

for Movement Disorders

Rebuilding Strength, Balance and Flexibility for Parkinson's Disease and Dystonia

Revised Edition

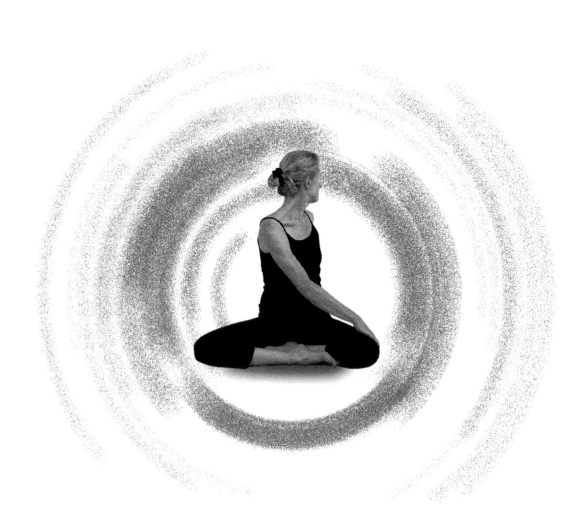

YOGA
for Movement Disorders

Rebuilding Strength, Balance and Flexibility for Parkinson's Disease and Dystonia

Revised Edition

Renée Le Verrier, RYT

Foreword: Lewis Sudarsky, MD
Director, Movement Disorders Clinic, Brigham & Women's Hospital
Associate Professor of Neurology, Harvard Medical School

My gratitude to the students and teachers I've had the opportunity
to share yoga practice with; I learn from each of you.

Renée Le Verrier, RYT

Caution: As with any exercise program, check first with your doctor before practicing the
poses presented here. Better yet, show your doctor this book so that he or she can see
specifically what you'd like to do. There are precautions for osteoporosis, hip replacement,
high blood pressure and glaucoma, as well as other conditions. Your doctor can advise you.

ISBN 978-0-9853869-1-7

Photographs by Andrew Edgar

Design & Artwork by

SMK Design

HoneyDew Productions

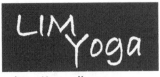

http://www.limyoga.com

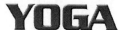
Contents

Foreword:
   Lewis Sudarsky, MD 7

Preface:
   Why Yoga? 8
   Revised Edition: The Science of Yoga 9

PART 1:
   Introduction 10

Chapter 1: The Path Home 11
   The Diagnosis 11
   My Yoga Journey .12
   The Prognosis 13
   Your Yoga Journey 13

Chapter 2: Before You Begin 14
   Beginning Your Practice 14
   Breathing 14
   Warm-ups and Poses 15
   When and Where .15
   What to Wear 16
   Props 16
   Format 18
   Asana Practice 18
   Coming to Stillness 18
   Warm-ups 18
   Poses 18
   Relaxation 19

   Especially Beneficial 21
   Yoga to Go: Applying It to Your Day 21
   Words of Caution .21
   Note to Teachers .22

Chapter 3: Warm-ups 24
   Preparation 24
   Breath 24
   Movement 25
   Set A 25
   Set B 37
   Variations 43
   Especially Beneficial 47

PART 2:
   Practice 48

Chapter 4: *Sunday:* Find Warmth 49
   Asana Practice 49
   Coming to Stillness 50
   Poses 50
   Relaxation 59
   Especially Beneficial 60
   Yoga to Go: Applying It to Your Day 60

Chapter 5: *Monday:* Know It Is There 62
   Asana Practice 62
   Coming to Stillness 63
   Warm-ups 63

Poses 63
Relaxation .74
Especially Beneficial. 74
Yoga to Go: Applying It to Your Day 75

Chapter 6: *Tuesday:* Twist It 76
Asana Practice 76
Coming to Stillness 76
Warm-ups 77
Poses 77
Relaxation .83
Especially Beneficial. 83
Yoga to Go: Applying It to Your Day 84

Chapter 7: *Wednesday:* Follow Your Breath 85
Asana Practice 85
Coming to Stillness 85
Warm-ups 87
Poses 87
Relaxation .89
Especially Beneficial. 89
Yoga to Go: Applying It to Your Day 90

Chapter 8: *Thursday:* Stay Strong 91
Asana Practice 91
Coming to Stillness 91
Warm-ups 92
Poses 92
Relaxation .101
Especially Beneficial. 101
Yoga to Go: Applying It to Your Day 101

Chapter 9: *Friday:* Flow 103
Asana Practice 103
Coming to Stillness 103
Warm-ups 104
Poses 104
Relaxation .111
Especially Beneficial. 112
Yoga to Go: Applying It to Your Day 112

Chapter 10: *Saturday:* Restore 113
Asana Practice 113
Coming to Stillness 113
Warm-ups 114
Poses. 114
Especially Beneficial. 122
Yoga to Go: Applying It to Your Day 122

Chapter 11: Meditation and More 124
Beginning Your Practice 124
When and Where. 125
Props. 125
Techniques .126
Especially Beneficial. 127
Meditation to Go: Applying It to Your Day. 127

Bibliography. 128

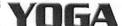

Foreword

Patients with a neurologic disease can regain some of the mobility they have lost through an exercise program. Le Verrier has put together an instructional guide to yoga with neurologic patients in mind. It is a clear, illustrated text which also touches on her personal journey. Yoga can be the cornerstone of a rehabilitation program for patients with Parkinson's disease, dystonia, and other movement disorders. These exercises also benefit patients with other neurologic problems. This is a graduated approach, but check with your doctor before you embark to ensure that these exercises are appropriate for you.

If you have Parkinson's disease, it's not your fault. We don't presently know the cause or causes of this complex disorder. It is generally considered to be due to a variety of genetic and environmental factors. There is, however, a great deal you can do to optimize your function and minimize the disability related to this disease. These exercises provide benefits to patients with movement disorders which help restore function and complement the effects of medication. Exercise is often as important as medication in getting back some of the motor control that Parkinson's disease has compromised.

People have different goals in mind beginning an exercise program. Some people exercise to improve muscle strength. Some people seek to improve endurance, to expand the capacity of the heart and lungs. These exercises work on flexibility and postural control, which are particular problems for patients with Parkinson's disease and dystonia. Yoga is good for the body as well as the spirit. With practice and teaching, we can all achieve better posture and a more natural manner of movement. When we move through life more effectively, we feel better.

Lewis Sudarsky, MD
Director of Movement Disorders Clinic, Brigham & Women's Hospital
Associate Professor of Neurology, Harvard Medical School

Preface

Why Yoga?

'[Yoga students] are really happy with who they are. and they bring a spirit of acceptance – not acceptance of their limitations. but of who they are in the world,.
– Peggy Cappy

Movement disorders such as Parkinson's disease affect more than the body. They leave a mark on our emotions, sometimes our mental capacity, often our whole spirit.

Tremors, rigidity, and imbalance invade us physically. As a result, our emotions are held captive. Fear – of falling, of the progression of the toxin in our brains or that another blood vessel will burst, of losing so much – takes over our thoughts. Then, there's struggle. The simplest movements – the dexterity needed to uncap the toothpaste or hold the spoon steady enough to eat a cup of soup – are monumental challenges that erode our ability to stay positive.

Moving through the poses and flows of yoga helps reduce muscle rigidity and increases strength, balance and flexibility. Yoga also affects more than the body; it balances our emotions, calms our mind, and creates peace in our spirit.

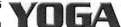
Preface
Revised Edition
The Science of Yoga

'Yoga helped older stroke victims improve balance. endurance,
– Indiana University study

'Yoga reduces fatigue in multiple sclerosis patients,
– Oregon Health & Science University study

Until recently, claims that yoga practice benefits those of us living with a movement disorder derived from those of us living with a movement disorder. Science, however, is catching up. Research now reveals that yoga is a beneficial therapy for conditions such as Parkinson's, stroke recovery and MS.

In a study conducted by the Parkinson's Disease and Movement Disorder Society of India, the findings showed "significant improvements in mobility, emotional well-being and moods and quality of life in people with Parkinson's after yoga practice."

Further testing is being done based on the results of a pilot study at the Weill Cornell Medical Center linking yoga with "increased energy, improved sleep, and reduced stress and stiffness in participants."

Researchers at Kansas University discovered "nice surprises" at the results of testing the physical benefits of yoga in people with Parkinson's. Tremor and fatigue were significantly reduced. An Indiana University research team found "exciting" results in their study on yoga's effect on stroke patients.

More studies are under way to support that we need not lose strength, flexibility and balance with a diagnosis. With them will be more proof to support the connection between yoga and improved health and well-being in people living with movement disorders.

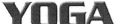
Part 1

Introduction

"I think I was most amazed by the visible reduction in tremoring and improvement in the steadiness of gait immediately following the yoga sessions."

Yvonne Searls, PT, PhD, Kansas University
The Therapeutic Effects of Yoga in Individuals
with Parkinson's Disease

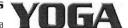
Chapter 1
THE PATH HOME

'Just tell the truth to yourself of what it is because
what is not acknowledged cannot be healed,.
– Lilias Folan

THE DIAGNOSIS

My symptoms confused the neurologists at first. They confused and terrified me too. A force was taking over my body. It was the tiger.

The tiger was my worst fear as a child. I was convinced that one would leap through my bedroom window while I slept. I lay on my bed peering at the curtain. It wasn't the summer breeze that made it flutter, it was tiger's breath. He was out there.

At the end of my eleventh summer, the tiger visited. I recognized him immediately, even though he didn't appear in his traditional black stripes or jump in through the window. He did, however, pounce and leave his mark.

This tiger was in my brain. I'd been born with an AVM – an arteriovenous malformation. A twisted mass of blood vessels, an AVM can linger undetected anywhere in the body. Until it bursts. I was in the eighth grade when it turned the left half of my body to lead. I'd had a stroke.

When I walked out of the month-long hospital stay, bald from the surgery, my left leg dragged behind. But with physical therapy, it gained some strength and balance. My right leg kicked in most of the effort and though I was anything but symmetrical, I hiked. I bicycled. I swam.

So, thirty-five years later, when my left leg started getting stiffer, less responsive, I again heard the tiger growl. Did I have another AVM? I also felt my right wrist and fingers lose coordination. Did I have two AVMs?

Neurologist number one diagnosed Parkinson's. He explained that the disease causes stiffness all over, affecting weak areas first. That explained the decrease in the use of my left leg. He added that disease itself was attacking the right arm and leg.

No. That would be just too cruel, even for a hungry tiger. I'd be out of sides. Parkinson's became a four-letter word. It wasn't spoken aloud in the house. If reference had to be made to it, we didn't say *Parkinson's*. We called it *The P-word*. I sought a second opinion. I sought any opinion that wouldn't pounce and take control over me.

Neurologist number two declared, Not The P-word. *Hooray.*

Clinging to number two's *Not*, I went neurologist-free for a year. My symptoms remained. Actually, they got worse. A tremor crept into my thumb. I stumbled.

Neurologist number three said it looked like a mild stroke. I can handle stroke, I thought. Did that, been there. Nice tiger. One recovers from a stroke. I voted for stroke. But symptoms canceled out my vote. I started moving in slow motion, lost my balance while standing at the dryer folding laundry.

Neurologists numbers four and five concurred: The P-word. My worst fear. The scariest tiger yet. Oh, string of four-letter words.

MY YOGA JOURNEY

Duane wore baggy sweats with oversized T-shirts. He taught at the Y. When I entered his class for the first time – my first time in any yoga class – he looked as though he'd be as comfortable on the couch with the TV remote as he did on the towel he used as a mat. I liked that. He didn't seem like he'd wrap his leg around his head in some advanced pose and expect the class to do the same. I really liked that.

I wanted a stretching class. We stretched. But we also breathed and became aware of sensations in our bodies. It was in his class that I first heard "Don't judge. Simply observe." *Don't judge?* Don't harangue my body for losing balance in tree pose? Don't frown for not being able to straighten my legs in down dog?

Duane's statement freed up a lot of brain space. I hadn't realized all the chatter going on up there. With his *Don't judge*, clouds floated away. If entering the Y's fitness room was my first step toward yoga, *Don't judge* was the long jump toward something bigger than just stretching. He had me connecting with my body, listening to what it said. By clearing the monologue in my head, I could hear so much more.

I was learning to rest comfortably in the present, instead of worrying about the past or fretting about the future. Any body, I discovered, even one with Parkinson's, can find that calm abiding place. When I'm there, I'm not saddened by loss because the past is truly behind me. When I'm there, I'm not afraid because my fears are *what ifs* of the future. When I'm there, I'm truly here.

Teaching and practicing yoga has given me strength. My arms, legs and core abdominal muscles all carry me straighter and with more ease. I've discovered my balance has improved. And even when my medication dose wanes, I'm not as rigid. The inner strength and balance I've gained has also led me to witness what is and accept it. At times, even

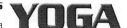
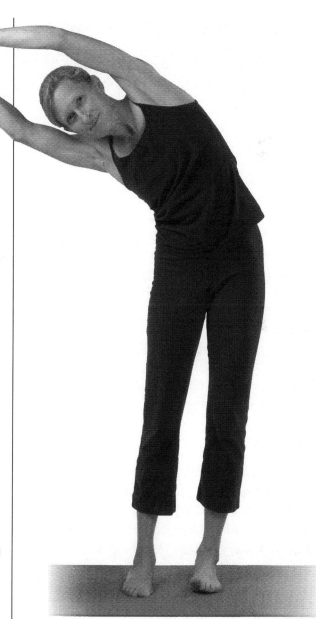

embrace it. I'm becoming as comfortable in my body as Duane looked in his that first day.

THE PROGNOSIS

I say it aloud now. *Parkinson's*. I can even put it in the same sentence with "I" and "have." But it doesn't have me. It is through yoga – its poses, self-reflection, living in the present – that I've learned to no longer fear the tiger. Oh, it's still here. But it doesn't pounce or take control anymore. I've tamed him and we live side by side.

YOUR YOGA JOURNEY

Living with a movement disorder is a challenge. The array of symptoms and the prognosis for cures can bring fear, struggle and loss of spirit, derailing our emotions, relationships, life as it was. In addition, the physical hurdles – stiffness, facial tics, rigidity, loss of balance, weakness, awkward movements – are there every day, every moment.

Whatever led to your diagnosis and wherever you are in living with your symptoms, practicing yoga can help you get back in balance emotionally and physically. The nonjudgmental, peaceful center of yourself is a healing place. Yoga is a path to that center. It won't cure the disorder, but it can bring you gently back to yourself.

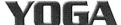
Chapter 2
BEFORE YOU BEGIN

'Wisely and slow. They stumble that run fast,
– Romeo and Juliet, William Shakespeare

In yoga practice, certain poses prepare us for other poses. Mind and body connect. And breath, movement, and a gradual turning inward all support one another.

It's like a crossword puzzle. The challenge is to find the working combination of letters to fit together across and down, playing off each other, one word supporting another.

BEGINNING YOUR PRACTICE

Each day as the week progresses, the *New York Times* crossword puzzles increase in difficulty. Beginners start with Monday's entry, filling in the answers in pencil. Within a couple of weeks, they might even try Tuesday's puzzle.

With practice, veterans get to know the common clues and grow to understand the nuance in others. They switch to using a pen. Over time, they sail through to Friday's grid, building up to the challenge of the weekend puzzles.

An ease-into-it approach to yoga is particularly beneficial when muscle rigidity and balance are of concern. For those of us with movement disorders, overworking rigid muscles can cause spasms. Stretching too far can damage a tendon. Coming into and out of a pose with too much force can cause dizziness, an injury or a fall. This is yoga where less is more.

Begin wherever you are. Each time you sit on the chair or step onto the mat, consider it a new time. Medications may be "on" one day and not the next. Perhaps you experienced a solid night's sleep one night but woke at 3:00 a.m. another. Begin each practice with where you are at that moment.

BREATHING

In yoga, movement follows the breath. Literally, we start with simply the breath. We bring our awareness to it and allow it to guide us inside with it. In noticing our breath, we center ourselves by releasing all the busy thoughts, releasing tension and worry along with them.

We also follow the breath when we begin to move. Typically, we exhale into a pose and inhale coming out of the pose, allowing the body to flow with the

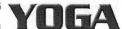
wave of our breathing. The steps for each of the poses note if the movement is done on an inhale or exhale. Most importantly, breathe fully and follow your rhythm of breathing. If your breath is strained, your body is likely to be, too.

WARM-UPS AND POSES

Begin simply. Start with the warm-ups in Chapter 3 and practice a few at a time. Get to know them, in your mind and in your body. Add a few more to your practice and then include a few steps from one of the chapter's list of poses, alternating days for variety. If you begin to struggle, take a break.

A difficulty description appears below each set of poses in Chapters 4 through 10. In most chapters, there are seated and standing variations of the same flow. The seated variation works most, if not all, of the same muscle groups as the standing variation, but with the stability of sitting on a chair.

It is helpful to move through the seated option first, even if you're able to try the standing version. This lets your muscles get a sense of the stretches at a base level. Once you're standing, stay near the chair to reach out for the chair back for support at any time. I've found I feel safe using a chair both seated and for support when standing. I can stretch with better alignment and more deeply because I'm not worried about losing my balance.

If you're new to yoga, welcome. If you've practiced yoga before and you're returning to it, welcome back. Take pleasure easing into it.

WHEN AND WHERE

What is the ideal setting for practicing yoga? Unlike a crossword puzzle where only one answer fits, there are many options for when and where yoga can fit into your day. Select a time that is quiet and the most comfortable space for you and your schedule.

It's a good idea to wait at least an hour after eating before doing any *asanas*, or poses. Many find that early morning practice works best, before breakfast but after the first round of my medication. Whatever time you decide, schedule an extra half hour on either side so you're not rushed to begin or end.

An hour is a standard length of a yoga class. Some are forty-five minutes, some up to two hours. The flows in this book vary but on average take about an hour. If you have more time, take an extra few minutes at the beginning and end on the opening breathing practice and closing guided imagery. If you have less time, flow through fewer poses. The Coming to Stillness and Relaxation aspects of the practice are as beneficial as the asana practice. So, with limited time you can move from breathing exercises directly to relaxing in savasana.

Another option is to pepper your practice through the day. Ten minutes in the morning to start your day can be followed by another ten-minute afternoon break. Evening presents an opportunity for ten minutes or more of relaxing, forward-bending poses that help invoke sleep.

Select a room that is comfortable and as free from distractions as possible. When you set up your mat and chair, be certain there are no end tables or other obstacles near enough to injure you if you fall. Consider setting up near a wall for an additional place to reach out to for balance should you need it. If transferring to a chair is difficult, you can sit on the edge of your bed. Place a folded towel or small pillow under your sitting bones so your hips are level or tilted forward slightly and not curving down into the bed.

Consider personalizing your space with candles, flowers or a memento that is meaningful to you. Each time you step on the mat or sit on the chair, you'll know you're somewhere special.

WHAT TO WEAR

Clothes that allow you to move and stretch work best for yoga. Opt for elastic or drawstring waistbands rather than snaps and zippers. Avoid buttons in tops as they may dig into your skin in a reclined position. Also, tops that are too loose can both get in the way when twisting and slip over your head when bending forward.

There's no need to purchase special pants and tops. The main reason many yoga teachers and students don yoga pants and sports tops is that they are form-fitting. This not only keeps excess fabric out of the way, it allows for observation. When a teacher demonstrates a pose, the students can see the positioning better than if the instructor is wearing a baggy outfit. The same holds true for the teacher being able to see if the student is in a safe position when in a pose, and not, for example, overextending a knee.

Try to practice barefoot. The sensation of the mat on the bottom of our feet helps with balance and you'll get more traction in standing poses, which will prevent injury from slipping. Besides, it gives your toes some freedom. It is, however, okay to practice with your shoes on, especially if you have special supports or braces in them that help you balance.

PROPS

Movement disorders throw us out of alignment, whether from one-sided weakness, muscle rigidity, slow movement, or spasms. Alignment is an essential factor in yoga. Joints function at their best when lined up properly with good blood flow. Nerves don't get pinched and energy moves. Proper alignment also prevents injury from overstretching or straining areas that don't move freely.

I haven't been symmetrical since the seventh grade. But I can be with props. Props help where we need straightening. Sitting on the edge of a cushion, for example, can put your hips in a neutral position, lengthening your back without strain. Light weights such as sandbags or sacks of rice help calm tremors, allowing an arm to relax instead of curl up with tension.

Yoga props

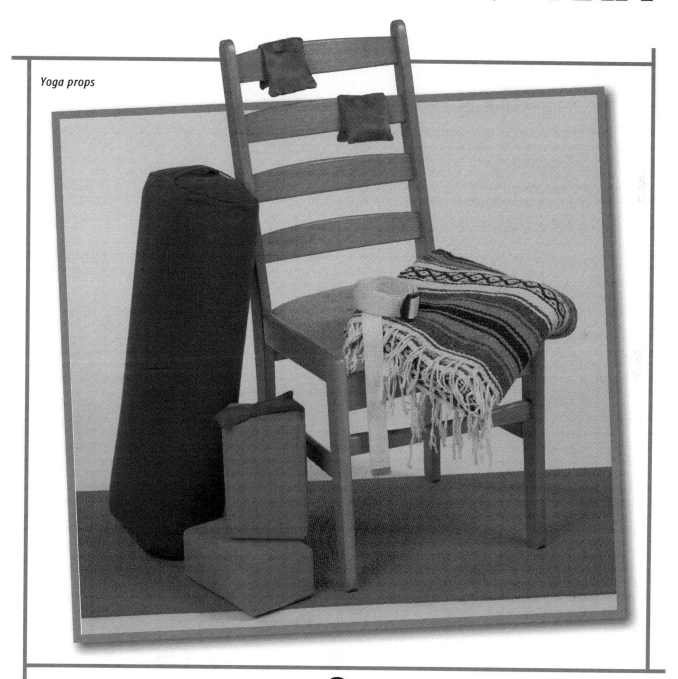

A chair not only raises the floor closer to your upper body, it provides stability when sitting or standing. Blocks also bring the floor closer so you won't strain your back or hamstrings reaching for the floor. A book or stack of books can substitute for blocks.

Bolsters provide support in reclining positions. Sofa cushions make good bolsters. Straps can be used to support, by giving added length to your arms when you can't reach. Use a webbed cloth belt in lieu of a yoga strap.

The mat itself, often called a "sticky mat," prevents slipping. Using props can make the difference between a healthy yoga practice and one fraught with injury.

FORMAT

Part 1 prepares you for practicing yoga. Part 2 presents a daily guide to yoga practice. The chapters flow as a yoga class does, with an initial centering or calming few moments followed by warm-up movements that lead to the poses. The practice ends with relaxation.

There are two additional segments that highlight the particular benefits of the poses and that suggest ways to carry your yoga practice into the rest of your day.

ASANA PRACTICE

Coming to Stillness

These few moments allow for the transition from what you were doing before yoga to your practice. The focus is on breath work, which helps bring your awareness – from the day's tasks or pondering what's for dinner – back to yourself. This allows your mind to connect to what's going on in your body, bringing you into the present moment.

Warm-ups

Chapter 3 details the warm-up poses. Begin with the warm-ups. Don't skip them. They're good for you. They're fat-free, dairy-free, gluten-free, and will help keep you injury-free. Take it slowly. Yoga is a wonderful tool but not a quick fix.

Poses

The week brings you full circle. Like moving from sunrise to sunset, the full seven days cover calming, strength, balance, flexibility, and relaxation poses.

Each chapter revolves around a theme for that day. Sunday focuses on the sun, with sun salutations. Monday introduces the moon series. Tuesday describes the benefits and how-to steps of twists while Wednesday covers breathing exercises and why they're so beneficial. Thursday's asana practice works on building strength and balance and Friday pulls it

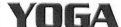
all together in a series of poses that flow from one to the next. Saturday, the traditional day of rest, invites you into restorative poses.

Relaxation

Yoga classes routinely end with a final pose called *savasana*, which translates as the corpse pose. It is a restful several minutes – preferably twenty but at least ten – where you lie comfortably and let go of thoughts and active movement and allow your body to absorb the benefits of the poses. The longer and deeper the relaxation, the better it is for the body because healing occurs when we are in this state of ease.

Each chapter ends with a guided relaxation to help lead you into the restful pose of savasana. Transitioning into this relaxed pose involves easing down onto the mat and arranging your blankets or bolsters. The Variations section in Chapter 3 suggests how to get down onto the floor using a chair. If you find it difficult to get down onto the floor, you can raise your legs onto another chair. You can also have your chair positioned near a bed or couch so you can put your feet up.

Take a few minutes to be sure you're comfortable, whether you're on the floor or in a chair. Reposition if you need to so that you'll be comfortable for the

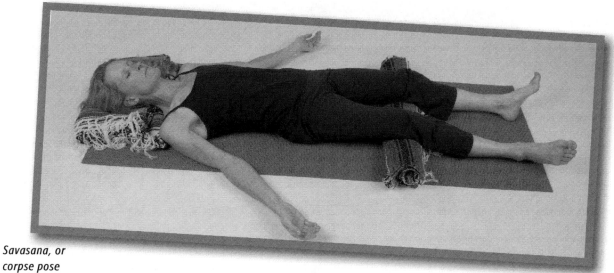

Savasana, or corpse pose

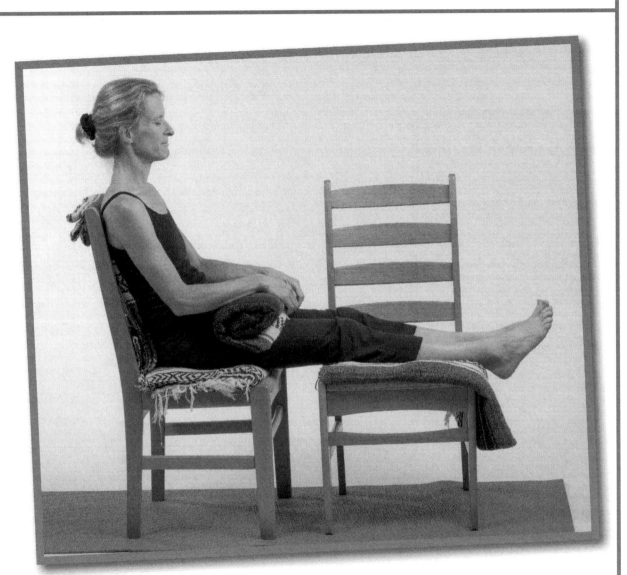

Savasana on chairs

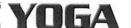
full ten to twenty minutes. Consider covering up with a blanket. Our bodies cool down without movement, and it is difficult to fully relax if you get chilled.

It is helpful to have someone read the guided imagery pieces to you. Or, you may want to record yourself reading the guided pieces to play during Savasana.

As important as settling into savasana is coming out of it. Take your time transitioning from this final pose. If you have blood pressure issues, whether they stem from symptoms or the side effects of medication, consider Savasana on the chair. In either case, open your eyes slowly. Stand up with care. Let the relaxed state stay with you.

ESPECIALLY BENEFICIAL

This list follows the asana practice and highlights the aspects of the poses that are of particular help in alleviating symptoms of movement disorders. It mentions muscle groups as well as functionality of a certain area.

YOGA TO GO: APPLYING IT TO YOUR DAY

This final list suggests ways to continue your yoga after you've rolled up the mat. Simply being aware of your breath at times throughout the day brings your mind and body together. These ideas aim at creating that connection in everyday living.

WORDS OF CAUTION

CHECK WITH YOUR DOCTOR

As with any exercise program, check first with your doctor before practicing the poses presented here. Better yet, show your doctor this book so that he or she can see specifically what you'd like to do. There are precautions for osteoporosis, hip replacement, high blood pressure and glaucoma, as well as other conditions. Your doctor can advise you.

BE SAFE

If you're not confident about your balance, practice with a chair. Be sure all four legs of the chair are on a sticky mat to prevent sliding. Place your chair away from end tables and anything else that might cause injury if you fall from the chair.

Use the chair for support. Pause at any time you feel you need a rest. Ease up at any time you feel pain. Stop at any time you feel dizzy. Smile any time you feel good.

TAKE YOUR TIME

Some poses are simple to move in and out of with little effort or time. Others need you to take them slowly. All are most beneficial when approached with focus and awareness.

Ladder grams are word puzzles that can be deceptively easy. They list a beginning and end word.

By changing one letter in the first word once for each of a number of steps, you arrive at the end word. Some are quick games that need only three or four steps. Most are more challenging and take more time and concentration.

Rebuilding strength, flexibility and balance from weak and stiff muscles caused by a neurologically-based disorder can't be done quickly. The poses and exercises in this book will help you move toward strength and flexibility. Like a ladder gram, moving from *rigid* to *fluid* will take more than a few simple steps.

NOTE TO TEACHERS

SAFETY

If you're using chairs in your class and have students with balance concerns, please space the chairs out. Try to keep them ten feet from each other. In case someone does lose their balance, another person is less likely to be affected. Also, be sure that all four legs of the chair are on the mat during practice to prevent slippage.

Some symptoms of movement disorders affect cognition. The first few minutes after a deep relaxation can increase any confusion. If you can, incorporate an additional five or ten minutes after savasana for business updates – schedule changes and such – or a discussion or a social time to allow for the transition. This is helpful for those who drove themselves as well as for anyone waiting for a ride. Please make an extra mental note to be sure each student has a way home after class.

POSES

Modifications

If you plan to teach the modified poses in this book, practice them yourself and sense the energy of each, the standing and the sitting variations. Know them. Don't simply move into them, feel them. Note how the movement feels in your body.

Remember that it feels different in your students' bodies. While this is true for any yoga instruction, it is particularly so when working with people with movement disorders because nerve connections and pathways work differently. They're blocked or triggers cause involuntary rather than voluntary movement. You can't know what's happening in their bodies. You can, however, as you would with any student, observe and listen. Learn from them and modify these poses as you need to for your students.

Unlike "Slow Flow" or "Gentle" yoga, the aim of yoga for movement disorders is not to move through asanas slowly. Fluidity may be better achieved through strengthening or dance-like poses. To best match the needs of a student, consider not the ending position of the pose but rather the main

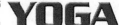
intent of the pose. Whether it's restorative, a twist or a shoulder opener, step through it. Move through one plane at a time. Perhaps flowing in and out of a chair-supported set of the first two steps successfully releases or strengthens an area.

Sequencing

Flowing in and out of poses is more beneficial to a student with a movement disorder than is holding a pose for any length of time. Holding a pose can trigger involuntary muscle contraction, spasms and overheating. Move and allow for resting breaths, which is a healthy approach on or off the mat.

STUDIO, CLASS OR HOME SETTING

For safety and comfort, try to arrange the environment so there are benches or chairs to sit on when a student arrives. Sitting down is often a necessity in order to remove shoes.

Clear any throw rugs or loose mats from the entry area. These are easy to trip over and can be a challenge to navigate around.

Consider keeping old mats on hand to use on studio floors for those who do not wish to remove their shoes. Orthotics, specially made shoes and certain soles help with gait and balance for some people and their asana practice could benefit from keeping their shoes on.

Fear of falling is prevalent among those of us with movement disorders. Creating a safe place to practice allows students to truly experience the benefits of yoga.

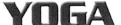
Chapter 3
WARM-UPS

'**Warm:** to infuse with the feeling of love,
friendship, well-being, or pleasure
up: in or into a better or more advanced state,
– **Merriam-Webster's Collegiate Dictionary**

The kitchen clock read 8:47 and morning yoga started at 9:00. I tossed my mat in the car rushed along the shortcut to class. Hardly anyone drove those back roads so I thought I'd make it in time. That day, the one vehicle on the same route appeared in my rear view mirror with its blue lights flashing.

I think back on being stopped for hurrying to yoga. I don't remember why I ran so late. I do remember missing most of class both because of my late arrival and because my mind kept reviewing me pulled over to the side of the road rather than me breathing into poses and savasana. The memory reminds me that preparing for yoga practice begins well before I step onto my mat or get seated on my chair.

PREPARATION

Warming up loosens tight areas, but that is only part of the process. We're also quieting our minds from the daily race to get somewhere so we can bring our attention to where we are at the moment. As we invite our awareness into our bodies, we learn to see what's going on in there. We notice what's calling out for attention, what's settling down. Physically, it keeps us in touch with our muscles and joints so we're less likely to overstretch, strain, or overheat. Mentally, this focus returns us to the present.

BREATH

The tool we use to bring our mind's attention to the body is our breath. We allow the breath to lead our focus inside. We also focus on the physical aspects of our breath by moving with our inhales and exhales. As the practice becomes more familiar, moving with the breath will become natural. And you may discover that this breath/motion connection creates more ease in moving through daily activities.

Begin from a comfortable seated position on a cushion or a straight-backed chair. Bring your attention to your breath. Follow it from the tip of your nose down into the base of your lungs. Let your ribs, front and back, expand. Feel them contract as you exhale. On the next inhale, notice the expansion up in the space between your shoulder blades. Feel the exhale releasing and relaxing them down your back. After several cycles of breath, move into warm-ups, Set A.

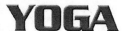
MOVEMENT

Work through Set A in order. Notice how your body feels after each warm-up. It may be enough for you physically or time-wise to stop after the set. Or, continue into the poses of any of the daily flows.

The poses in Set A bend, stretch, flex and rotate the spine in all the directions it's meant to move. Set B works specific areas. The chapters in Part 2 indicate which pose from the second set to add to your routine for the day's practice. You can also choose one or more on your own to do during any day of your practice.

At any time throughout the warm-ups, if you need to take a break, please do. Pause and take a resting breath. Mentally scan your body from head to toe and notice what's going on – aches, pockets of mobility that weren't previously there, a shift, no shift at all. In following my first teacher, Duane's advice, *Don't judge*. Simply notice.

SET A

Need: Straight-backed chair, Sticky mat

1. **SEATED MOUNTAIN**

a. This is the base pose for starting any seated position. It is quite active considering it looks as though we're simply sitting on a chair.

b. Sit at the front edge of your chair, your feet about hip width apart on the mat and your weight evenly balanced on both sitting bones, which are located at the center of each buttock.

c. Notice if your ankles are positioned directly below your knees, both making right angles.

d. Create space between your hips and your ribs, reaching upward but keeping your shoulders relaxed.

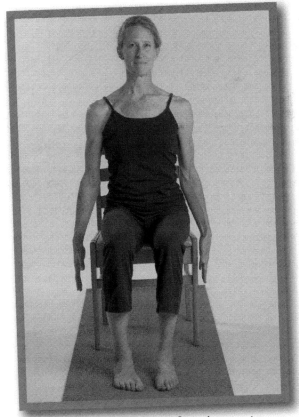

Seated mountain pose

e. Let your collarbones broaden as your shoulder blades slide down your back.

f. Lengthen up through the crown of your head, as though you're trying to touch the ceiling with the tassel of an imaginary hat.

g. If it's comfortable, let your arms drop to your sides and reach slightly through to your fingertips. Instead, you can rest your hands on the tops of your thighs.

h. And breathe.

i. Begin each of the seated warm-ups with this pose.

2. NECK RELEASES

a. These invite joint fluids into the cervical disks and help release tension.

b. From seated mountain pose, inhale. As you exhale, drop your chin to chest.

c. On the next exhale, turn to look over your right shoulder. Inhale to center. On the next exhale, turn to look over your left shoulder.

d. Inhale your head back to center.

e. On an exhale, drop your right ear to your right shoulder. Return to center on an inhale. On an exhale, drop your left ear to left shoulder. Inhale back up.

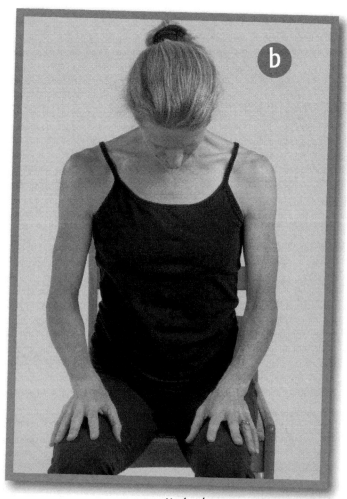

Neck releases

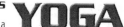
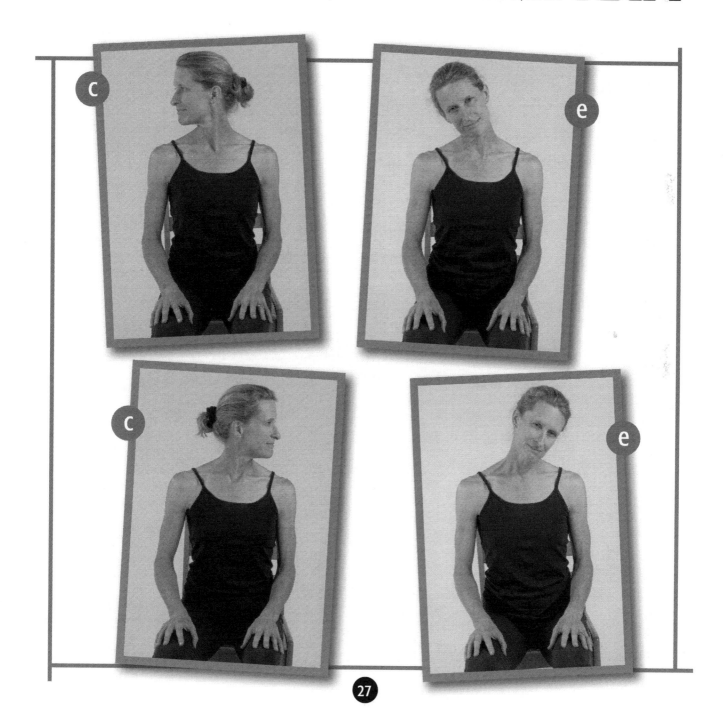

3. SHOULDER ROLLS

a. These unlock some of the many muscles and tendons that make up the shoulder.

b. Inhale and squeeze your shoulders up toward your ears, exhale and circle them back and around and down. Try this three times and reverse direction for three rounds. If more feels better, try a few more.

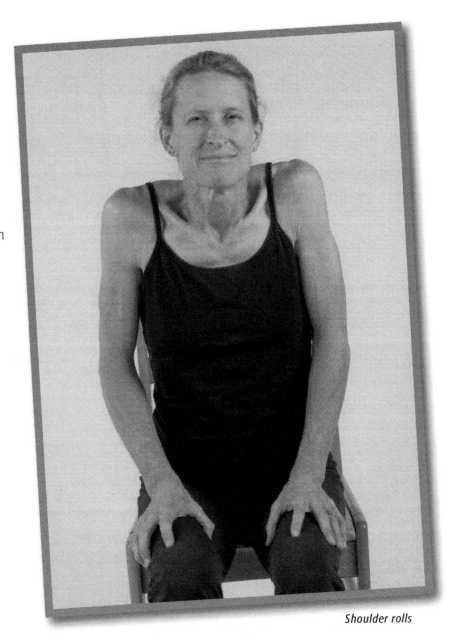

Shoulder rolls

4. WRIST STRETCHES

a. These coax blood into your fingers and free up some rigidity in the wrists.

b. Extend your arms in front of you, palms up. Take hold of your right fingertips with your left hand and on an exhale, press them toward the floor. Release and switch hands.

c. With your arms extended in front of you, turn your palms down. Take hold of your right fingertips with your left hand and on an exhale, press them toward the floor. Release and switch hands.

d. Release your hands back to your lap.

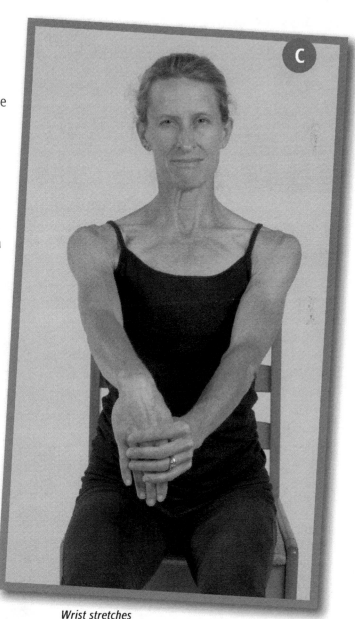

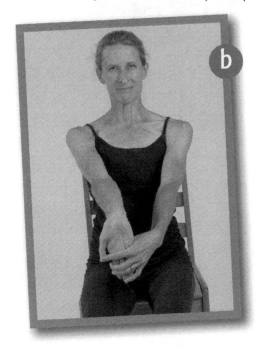

Wrist stretches

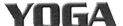

5. **UPWARD SALUTE**

a. This asana stretches the intercostals, the muscles between the ribs, opening up for full, deep breaths. It is also the beginning pose of a sun salutation, a way of greeting the day. I often take the opportunity in this pose to welcome what will come in the day, or state an intention for myself, such as *Stop and breathe – really breathe – today* or *Give a compliment today, maybe to someone else, maybe to myself.*

b. Drop your arms to your sides. Turn your palms out.

c. Feel the next inhale expand your chest and allow your arms to float up with that expansion, elbows straight and reaching through the fingertips. Note that if you see your elbows in front of you, reach higher to bring the insides of the elbows parallel to your ears. If it's comfortable for your neck, look up at your hands. If that causes strain, look forward or slightly above what is in front of you.

d. Turn your palms outward and allow an exhale to release your arms, lowering them down in big arcs.

e. Repeat two more times.

f. Note that if one arm is weaker, raise the stronger arm first and try using a strap, as noted in Variations at the end of this chapter.

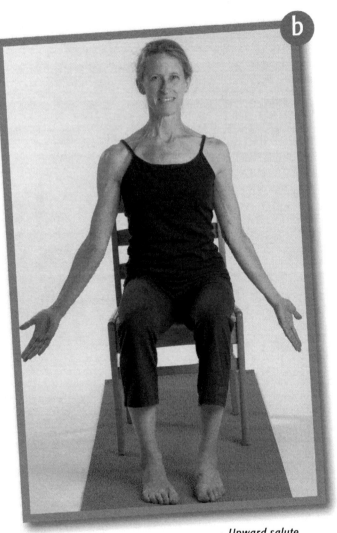

Upward salute

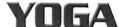
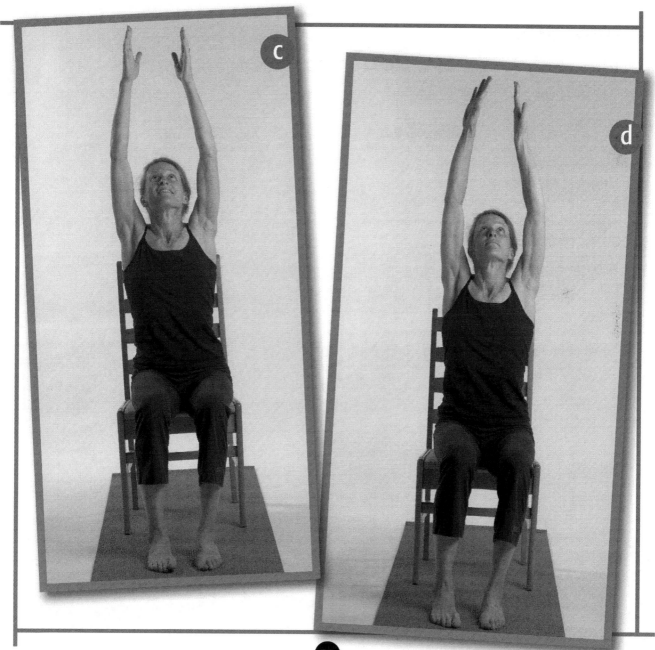

6. LATERAL STRETCH

a. This is another stretch for the intercostals as well as muscles in the hip and shoulder.

b. Drop your arms to your sides. For support, place your left hand on the chair seat beside your left hip.

c. Inhale and raise your right arm to the ceiling, your upper arm beside your right ear. At the same time, press down into the chair with your right sitting bone.

d. Exhale and reach the right hand to the left.

e. Inhale your arm to straight overhead and exhale it down to your side.

f. Repeat for the left side.

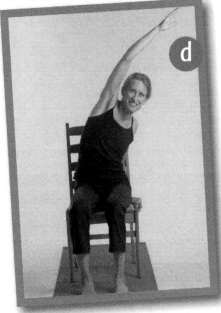

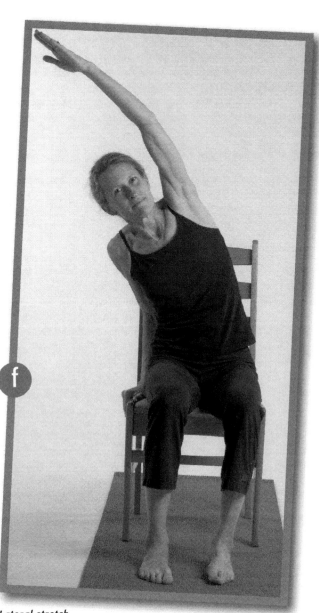

Lateral stretch

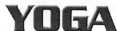
7. CAT AND DOG

a. These flex and extend the vertebrae of the spine and help soften rigidity in the torso.

b. Place your palms on your thighs. Inhale, and with an exhale, feel your belly squeeze in. Follow that motion by pressing your spine toward the back of the chair. Allow your shoulder blades to separate, round your shoulders forward and drop your chin to your chest.

c. Inhale and feel the belly expand, following that opening by pressing your navel forward, lifting your sternum up slightly, then allowing your shoulders to drop back.

d. For two more cycles of breath, exhale into cat, rounding your spine, and inhale into dog, arching your spine.

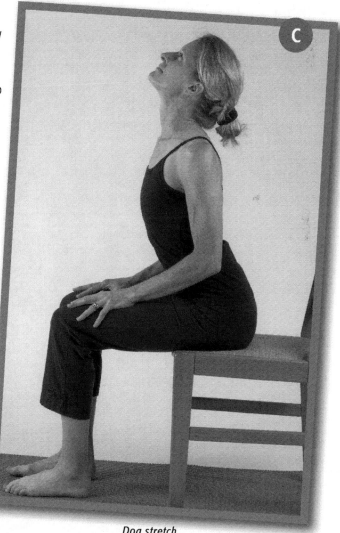

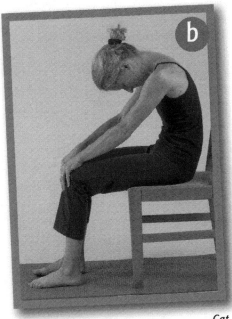

*Cat
stretch*

Dog stretch

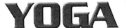
8. TWIST

a. Place your left hand on the outside of your right knee. Place your right hand on the chair behind your right hip.

b. Place enough weight onto your right sitting bone to free up your left hip so it can move with the twist.

c. Inhale and lengthen straight up.

d. With the exhale, twist your belly to the right.

e. Lengthen up with your inhale. On the exhale, twist your rib cage to the right.

f. Lengthen up with your inhale. On the exhale, turn your shoulders to the right. If it's comfortable, look over your right shoulder.

g. Use your arms for extra leverage as needed.

h. Inhale as you gently uncoil. Rest your palms on your lap.

i. Repeat on the left side.

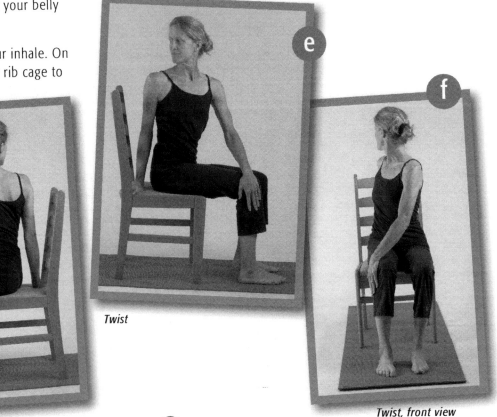

Twist

Twist, front view

9. **FORWARD BEND**

a. Beginning in seated mountain, take in a full breath and lengthen the spine. On an exhale, hinge forward at the hips. Maintain that lengthening out through the crown of your head while pressing the sitting bones down onto the chair.

b. Reach your palms toward the mat or on blocks beside your feet. Or, keep your palms on your thighs for support, protecting your lower back.

c. Follow the expansion of the next inhale by rounding back up into seated mountain.

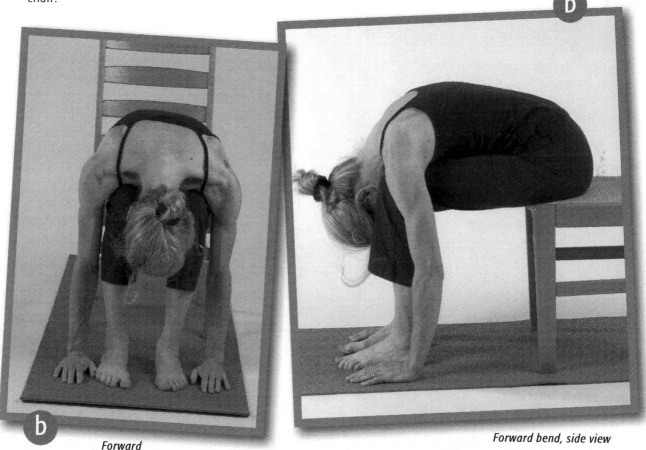

Forward bend

Forward bend, side view

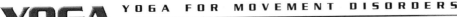

Shoulder opener hug

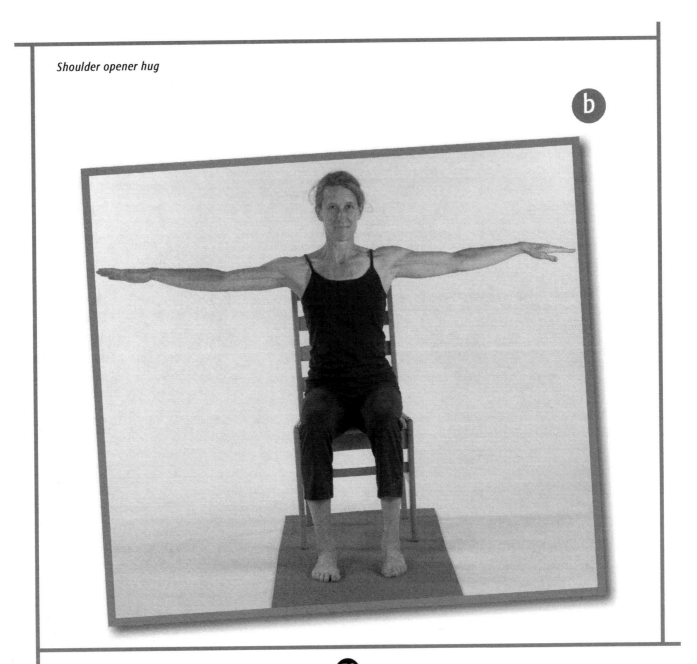

b

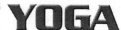

SET B

1. HUG

a. This opens the scapular area, or, the shoulder blades.

b. From seated mountain, extend your arms into a T position, reaching from your heart out through your fingertips.

c. Inhale, and on an exhale, bring your arms across your chest and wrap your hands around opposite shoulders. Notice which arm is on top.

d. On an exhale, turn your head to look over your right shoulder. Inhale back to center. Linger in the hug for a moment and note how it feels. On the next exhale, turn your head to look over your left shoulder.

e. Remembering which arm is on top, inhale back to a T position and repeat steps c and d with the other arm on top.

f. Release and bring your hands back to your thighs.

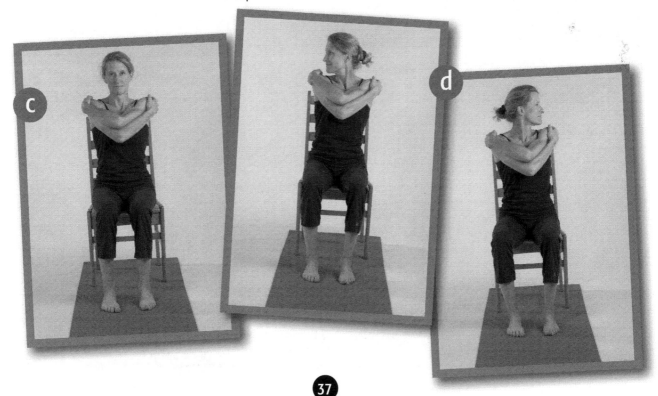

2. CIRCLE FROM HIPS

a. This lower back opener also releases the hips some.

b. Place your hands on your lap or at your waist.

c. Hinging at the hips rather than the waist, circle your torso clockwise, following your breath with the movement, coming forward with the exhales and circling back with the inhales. Reverse direction.

d. To keep your back straight as you circle, imagine a paintbrush at the top of your head and you're painting big circles on the ceiling.

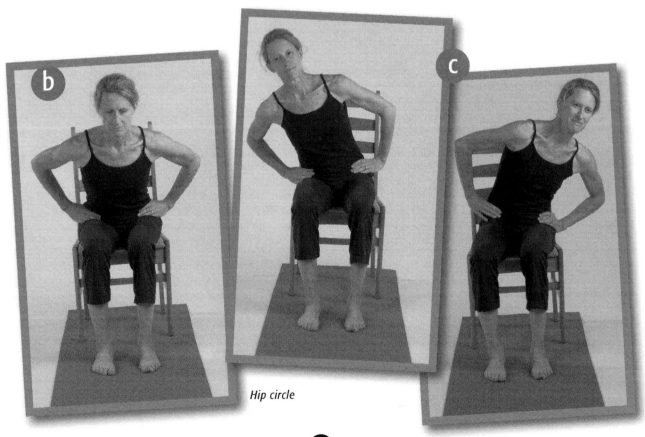

Hip circle

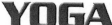
3. FOOT STRETCH

a. Oh, the forgotten feet. This stretches the many muscles in the arch, top of the feet and into the toes, which are so important for balance.

b. Position your feet as if you're standing on tiptoes, your foot as close as possible to a right angle to your toes. Begin by dropping the heel slightly then pressing down on tiptoes again. This not only loosens the ankle joint, the pumping motion can help with circulation.

c. Hold the tiptoe position for two rounds of breath.

d. Release and allow the left foot to be flat on the mat. Kick your right foot back, the top of your toes on the mat. Press into your foot slightly and hold the position for two rounds of breath.

e. Repeat for the left foot.

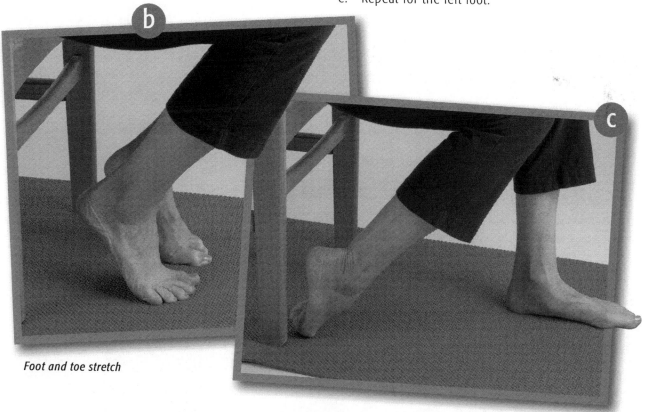

Foot and toe stretch

4. HEAD TO KNEE

a. This movement works the quadriceps in our front thighs and stretches the hamstrings in the back thighs. The extra bonus is that it also strengthens the abdominals. This is especially beneficial because the core muscles of the stomach and back carry us through when arms and legs are weak.

b. On an inhale, kick the right foot out, straightening that leg. Exhaling, bend your knee up towards your chest, rounding your back and reaching your arms around the bent leg.

c. Following the breath, repeat three more times.

d. Take a moment to notice how each leg feels before repeating with the left leg.

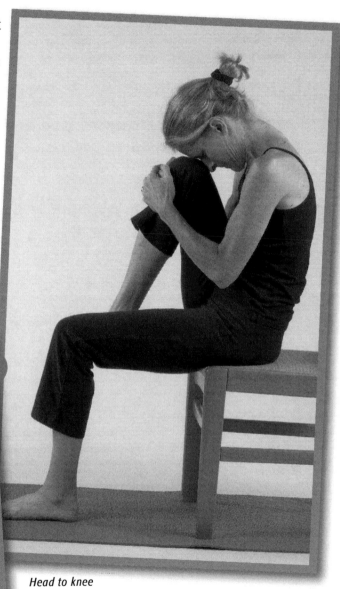

Head to knee

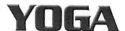

5. STANDING TWIST

a. If you're able to stand safely and comfortably, step behind your chair, several inches away. You can reach out for the chair back for support at any time. Be sure that all four legs of the chair are still on the mat.

b. Let your arms hang loosely at your sides. Swing from side to side, allowing your arms to follow the motion like empty coat sleeves. As your weight shifts onto your right leg, try to lift your left heel off the mat slightly so your left foot pivots a bit and keeps in line with your knee. Do the same with the right.

c. For more balance, hold onto the chair back with your right hand and twist your left arm to the left. As you swing baack to center, switch hands and twist your right arm to the right.

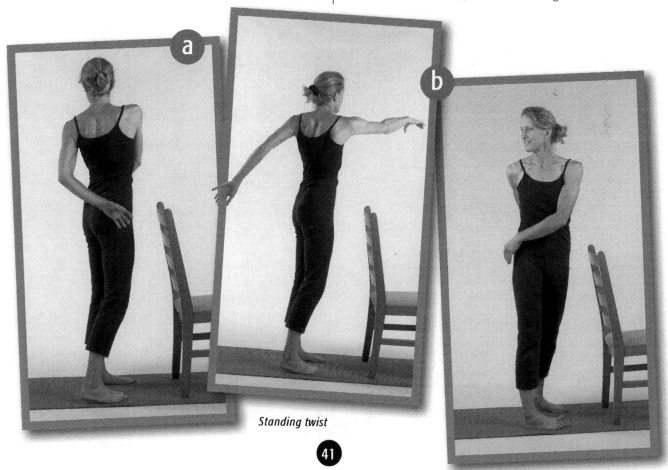

Standing twist

6. STANDING MOUNTAIN

a. This is the base pose for starting any standing position. It, too, like seated mountain, is an active pose.

b. Stand a few inches behind your chair, your weight evenly balanced on both feet. If you can, spread your toes wide. Feel the bottoms of your feet at the ball of your big toes as well as at the ball of your little toes. Notice the bottom of your heels on the inner as well as the outer edges.

c. Lift your kneecaps up by tightening your thighs. At the same time, try to pull your buttocks muscles down slightly.

d. Lengthen your spine by pressing up through the crown of your head, as though you're trying to touch the ceiling with the tassel of an imaginary hat.

e. Create space between your hips and your ribs, reaching upward but keeping your shoulders relaxed.

f. Try to broaden your shoulders. Raise your sternum, or breastbone, up toward the ceiling slightly, and tuck your chin slightly.

g. Let your arms drop to your sides and reach through to your fingertips.

h. And breathe.

i. Release and smile.

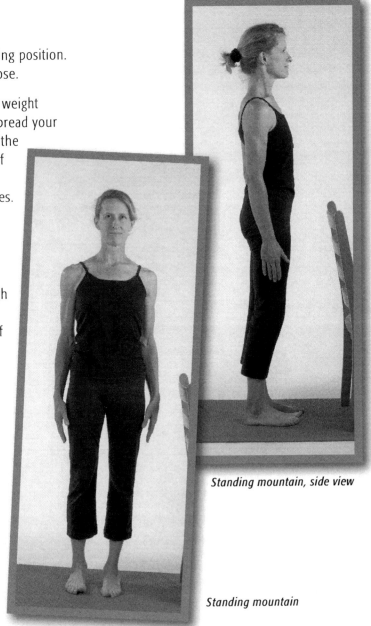

Standing mountain, side view

Standing mountain

VARIATIONS

I've often smiled to myself in a yoga class when the teacher asks us to notice how our right side and left side may feel different from one another. *May?* I can't remember when they felt the same.

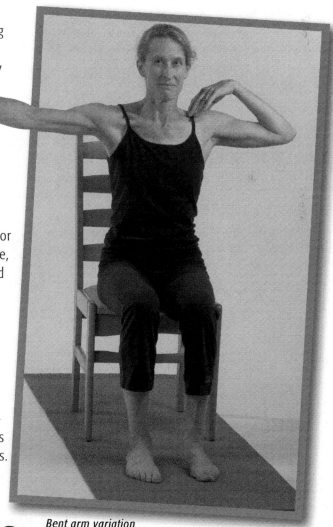

With many movement disorders, there's an imbalance, whether it's involuntary stiffness in one leg or an arm that doesn't respond quite as it should or has tremors or spasms. The imbalance or the intensity of it can differ from day to day based on medication cycles, the weather, sleep patterns. Adjust your yoga practice for where you are that day, even if that starting point bears no resemblance to yesterday's starting point.

Your body's cues tell you when to modify a pose or try a variation. These cues include strained breath or holding your breath, pain, fear of falling. If the steps for the pose say to lift both arms and you can lift only one, follow your body and lift only one. If you're concerned about balance, try the seated form of the pose. The variations that follow are suggestions for modifying.

Bend

If holding your arms out in a T position or raising them overhead triggers tremors or other involuntary movements, try bending that elbow. Also, if a straight-legged position causes spasms, try bending your knees slightly, taking the weight in your thighs, or quadriceps. Try moving gently between these positions, from straight elbow to bent or straightened knees to bent.

Bent arm variation

Strap

Straps, weights and blocks can help if you experience spasms in your legs or feet when seated. Sometimes, simply placing the soles of your feet on the floor triggers pressure points that cramp up toes or arches or cause such tension that your heels bounce involuntarily. Try calming this spasticity by strapping the heel to a block, or weighting the foot with a weight or sandbag or sack of rice.

Also, if your legs tend to flop to one side or the other while you're doing seated upper body poses, you can place a block between your knees. You could also add a strap above or below the knees, whichever is more comfortable for you.

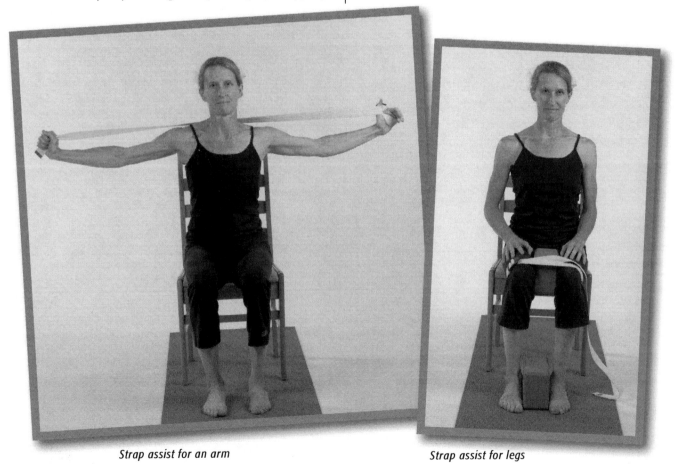

Strap assist for an arm   *Strap assist for legs*

Support

Moving down onto the mat can be a daunting task. But lying back brings a deeper relaxation during savasana and in the restorative poses in Chapter 10. Try using the chair, with some folded blankets for padding if needed, to ease your way down. Start with your chair on the mat to avoid slippage. Face the seat of the chair. Bend forward and place your hands on the edge of the seat and let your arms help you as you kneel onto the mat. Next, sink down to one hip and straighten your legs one at a time.

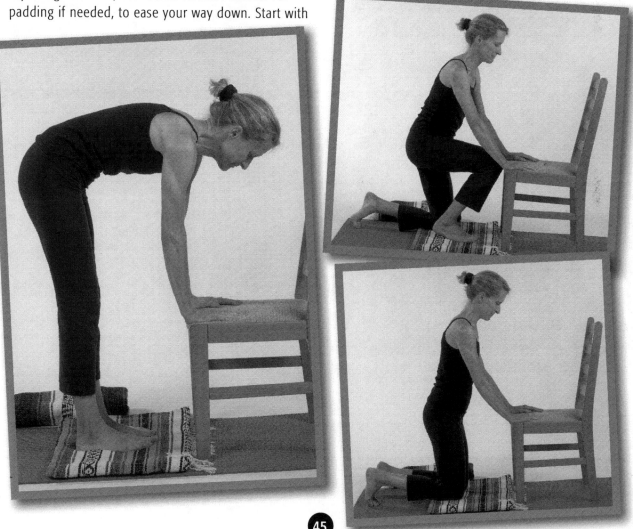

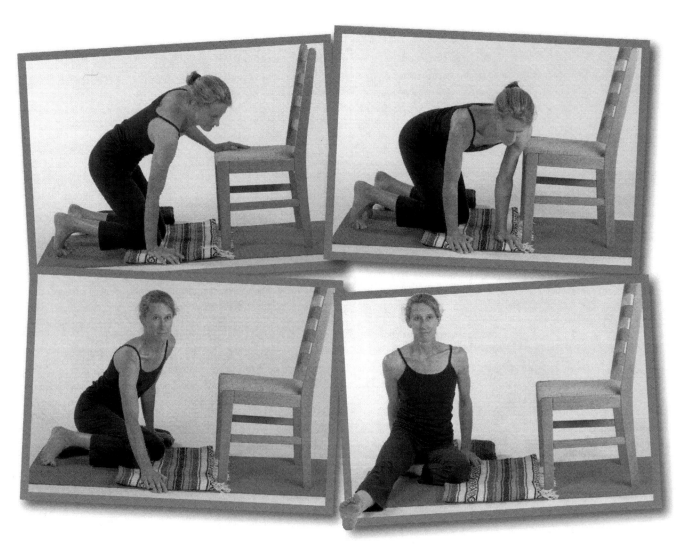

To get back to standing, bend your knees to one side and come up on your knees. Use the chair to help you rise up on your knees. Again, with your arms on the chair for support, bring one foot flat on the mat. For the best support and leverage to rise, try to position the ankle under the knee so that there are right angles at the ankle and knee. Bear weight on that leg and, using your arms for extra strength, begin to rise and bring the other leg forward as you straighten to standing.

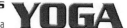
Lift

Wheelchair seats can put the spine in a rounded position. To straighten it and bring your hips into a neutral position, try placing a folded or rolled towel beneath your buttocks just behind your sitting bones. Another rolled-up towel placed down the length of your back can help as well.

ESPECIALLY BENEFICIAL

Tremors, medications, sleeplessness contribute to the fatigue that accompanies movement disorders. Seated or standing mountain pose, or tadasana, takes only a few minutes to move into, but the energizing effects of lining up our posture can last well beyond that time.

Mountain pose encourages body alignment, which helps maintain a more balanced gait.

YOGA TO GO: APPLYING IT TO YOUR DAY

Bringing our attention to our breath brings us into the present moment. We can practice this awareness in our warm-ups or at any time throughout the day.

Variations to poses help us gain the benefits of stretching or strengthening with less risk of falling or overdoing it. Are there aspects of your day that seem overwhelming? Try varying and modifying your approaches to them.

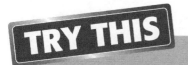

TENNIS ANYONE?

For those particularly knotty, stiff spots, try a tennis ball massage. Sit on a chair and roll one on the floor under your foot. Sit on the floor and roll your calf muscle back and forth over it. Hold it in one palm and gently roll it on the muscles of the other forearm.

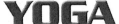
Part 2

Practice

"The results of the study showed a significant improvement in the group of individuals who underwent training in yoga classes....There was an improvement in their mobility, flexibility, emotional state as well as their quality of life."

Parkinson's Disease and Movement Disorder Society of India
The Efficacy of Yoga on Improving Quality of Life for Individuals with Parkinson's Disease

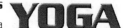
Chapter 4
SUNDAY: FIND WARMTH

'Give me the splendid silent sun...,
— **Leaves of Grass, Walt Whitman**

Naps happen, particularly on Sunday afternoons and especially in the winter in our house. Elsie curls up in her dog bed by a hot air grate, Billy Bird stands on his heated perch, and Scutes, the tortoise, basks beneath his sunlamp. The humans each find a sunny patch to settle into as well. A quiet warmth ensues. Whatever the season, it's a delicious way to begin the week.

ASANA PRACTICE

The sun salutation, or Suryanamaskar, is to many the heart of asana flows. Sun salutations work major joints, inviting synovial fluids that lubricate and cleanse. They also flex and extend the spine, creating warmth. In addition, sun salutations stretch and strengthen areas directly affected by movement disorders. These areas commonly become particularly stiff or rigid. They include the neck or cervical spine, scapular muscles around the shoulder blades, the thoracic or upper back spine and its surrounding muscles, hamstrings and calves in the back of the legs, hip flexors at the top front of the thigh as well as the joints of the shoulders, hips and ankles.

Accessibility marks another feature of sun salutations because they can be practiced standing on the mat or seated on a chair.

This versatile flow, as with many yoga poses, involves opposing forces – stretching up and down at the same time or simultaneously reaching forward and back. Yoga celebrates the balance within this duality. In sun salutations in particular, we greet the sun with open arms as well as bow down to the earth. The balance between this reach toward the sky and folding to the ground lies within us. We take on characteristics of each as we reside in the space between the sun and the earth.

If you need to take a resting breath during any of the steps of this asana, return to your mountain pose and bring your attention once again to the breath. As you move through this energizing flow, whether with or without pauses, allow yourself to recognize the sun's glow and the earth's solidity in your own radiance and strength.

Coming to Stillness

Find a comfortable yet straight-backed position on a cushion on the mat or on a chair, with your palms resting on your knees or with your hands on a pillow in your lap.

Notice your inhale and exhale in a full cycle of breath.

Let your eyes drift closed. Imagine you're outside on a cool, overcast day when, for a moment, the clouds dissipate and clear blue sky is unveiled.

Imagine a sunbeam shining on your face. Let it warm you, let it melt away the furrows in your brow and the clench in your jaw. Feel the heat on your skin and let your worries, your clouds, drift away.

Relax in your breathing and warmth for a few more cycles of breath.

Warm-ups

Chapter 3 for the ˙es to do before ʾowing flow. Work \ and pose 1

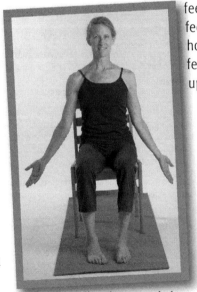

Sun salutation on a chair: upward salute

Poses

SUN SALUTATION

Seated Variation

> *Need: Straight-backed chair*
> *Sticky mat*
> *Blocks (optional)*

Difficulty: Any level can enjoy this version.

1. Sit in mountain pose.

2. **Upward salute**: Let your arms drop to your sides. Turn the palms out, and on an inhale, slowly raise both arms to the sky. If it feels comfortable on your neck and you feel stable, have a look up at the indoor horizon where ceiling meets wall. If you're feeling no neck strain, let your gaze move up and look at your fingertips.

   - As you exhale, allow your arms to open wide to the sun as you reach your arms back slightly, lifting your heart. This is a nice position to state an intention or affirmation to yourself, whatever it is that warms you today.

   - Inhale back to straight, arms still reaching to the sky.

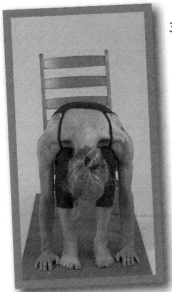

Forward bend

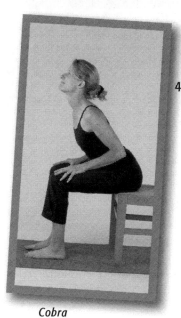

Cobra

3. **Forward bend**: Exhale as you slowly hinge forward at the hips, bowing to the earth. Keep your heart lifted as you fold forward. You can lower your arms to your thighs, or, if it feels comfortable, let your torso rest on your thighs. If there's no strain in your back or shoulders, allow your arms to straighten to the floor. Rest your palms flat on the mat or on blocks beside your feet.

4. **Cobra**: If your hands are on the floor, bring your forearms back to your thighs. On an inhale, put pressure into your forearms and push away from your thighs, bringing your head and shoulders up and forward. If it feels comfortable, lift your chin slightly.

5. Exhale and on an inhale, straighten back to seated mountain.

6. **Seated lunge**: Turn to sit sideways on the front edge of the chair. Bend the inside leg so the knee is at a right angle. Drop the outer leg, aiming the knee toward the mat. You can place a block, bolster or folded towel beneath this knee for comfort and support. On an inhale, lengthen up from the base of your spine out through the crown of your head.

7. Bring your legs and torso back to seated mountain facing forward.

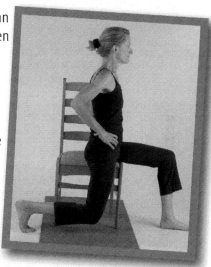

Lunge

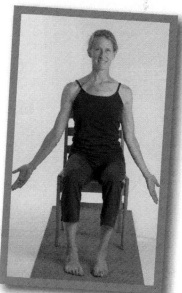

Upward Salute

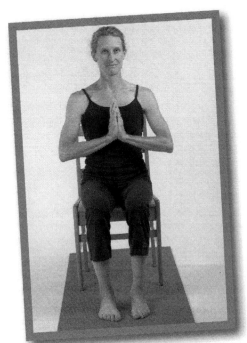

Namaste, seated

8. **Seated lunge**: Turn sideways on your chair facing the other way and repeat steps 6 and 7.

9. Turn to sit facing forward again. Inhale into an upward salute.

10. Exhale your hands down into prayer position over your heart.

11. Take a resting breath. Feel your heart with the backs of your thumbs. If you stated an intention or affirmation, this is a nice time to repeat it to yourself.

12. Move into the Relaxation that follows.

SUN SALUTATION

Chair-supported Variation
> *Need: Straight-backed chair*
> *Sticky mat*

Difficulty: The chair provides support, but this is still an energizing flow. If you're new to yoga and exercise or if you get overheated easily, try the seated variation first.

Place a chair on one end of your mat, the seat facing toward you as you stand in the center of the remaining mat. Be sure the legs of the chair are all on the mat, to prevent it from slipping.

1. Stand in mountain pose facing the chair, a few inches away from it.

2. **Upward salute**: Let your arms drop to your sides. Turn the palms out, and on an inhale, slowly raise both arms to the sky. If it feels comfortable on your neck and you feel stable, have a look up at the indoor horizon where ceiling meets wall. If you're feeling no neck strain, let your gaze move up and look at your fingertips.

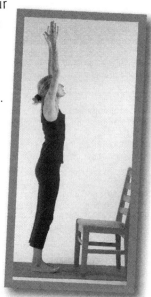

Sun salutation chair supported: upward salute

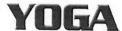
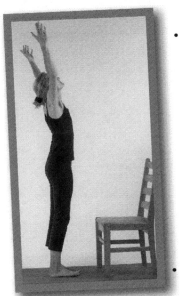

- As you exhale, allow your arms to open wide to the sun as you reach your arms back slightly, lifting your heart. This is a nice position to state an intention or affirmation to yourself, whatever it is that warms you today.

- Inhale back to straight, arms still reaching to the sky.

3. **Forward bend**: Exhale as you slowly hinge forward at the hips. Keep your heart lifted as you fold forward and drop your hands to the chair. Allow your knees to bend as generously as you need to for stability and so there is no strain on your lower back or hamstrings. Bow

Forward bend

your head. If it feels comfortable, let the crown of your head touch down lightly on the chair.

4. **Lunge**: Inhale and exhale as you step one leg back straight, bending your front leg.

- To prevent injury to your front knee, be sure your thigh and shin and your shin and foot are at right angles.

- Try to keep your weight even on both feet. If your hips become uneven side-to-side, try to level them out. Press the back heel toward the mat as you reach the front of the same hip toward the chair. Breathe.

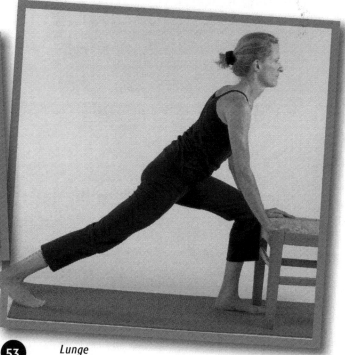

Lunge

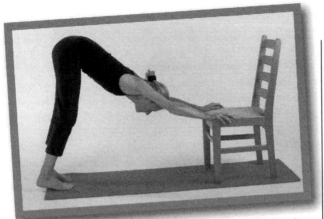

Downward-facing dog

5. **Downward-facing dog**: Exhale as you step your other leg back to meet the first one.

   • Press away from the chair with your hands and reach your tailbone back, hinging at the hips as your head drops so your ears are in line with your arms. Bend your knees slightly, or more if needed.

   • Keep pressing your tailbone back as you reach the crown of your head toward the seat of the chair.

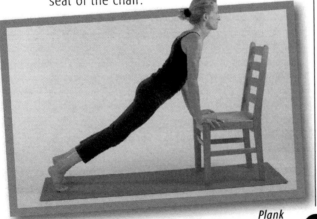

Plank

6. **Plank**: Inhale as you pull your hips and abdomen forward, letting your arms and feet bear the weight as your body straightens.

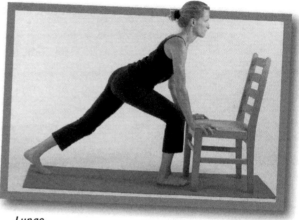

Lunge

7. Exhale back to downward-facing dog.

8. Inhale as you step one leg forward into a lunge. Exhale.

9. Inhale as you step the other leg forward into a forward bend. Bend your knees and press into the mat with your feet as you roll up into mountain pose.

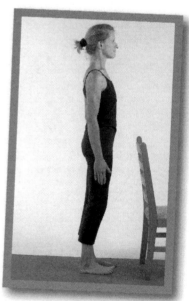

Mountain pose

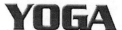
10. Inhale into an upward salute. Exhale your arms to your sides and take a resting breath in mountain pose.

11. Repeat Steps 1 through 3.

12. Repeat lunge in step 4 but reach back with the other leg this time, and continue through step 9.

13. Inhale into an upward salute.

14. Exhale your hands down into prayer position over your heart.

15. Take a resting breath. Feel your heart with the backs of your thumbs. If you stated an intention or affirmation, this is a nice time to repeat it to yourself.

16. Move into the Relaxation that follows.

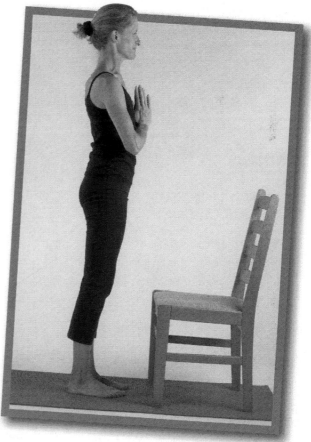

Upward salute

Namaste

SUN SALUTATION

Wall-supported Standing Variation

Need: Sticky mat

Difficulty: Challenging if you have balance concerns. Also, this is an energizing flow. If your symptoms include overheating or issues with body temperature regulation, try the seated variation listed before this. Please note: If you are avoiding forward bends, this may be a sun salutation that you can try because it does not include a forward bend.

Spread your mat so the short end is against a wall. Ideally, spread the mat near a corner where there's another wall arm's length away. This could help if you need to reach out for balance. If you're fearful of falling, please use the seated variation first.

1. Stand in mountain pose facing the wall, eight inches to a foot away from it.

2. **Upward salute**: Inhale as you slowly raise both arms to the sky, palms facing upward. If it feels comfortable and you feel stable, have a look up at your hands.

   - Exhale as you reach your arms back slightly, creating an arch in your upper back.

   - Inhale back to straight, arms still open to the sky. This is a nice position to state an intention or affirmation to yourself. I will

notice the sun today, or I shall be kind to myself today, or whatever it is that warms you today.

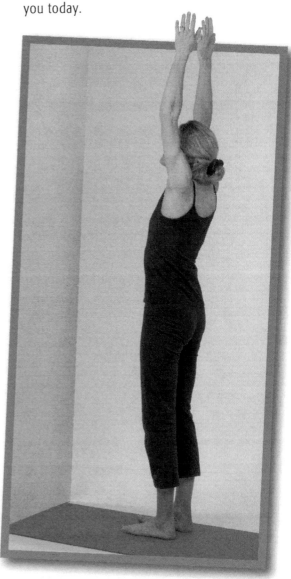

Sun salutation at wall: upward salute

3. **Lunge**: Exhale as you place your hands on the wall at shoulder level and step your right leg back straight, bending your front leg.

- To prevent injury to your front knee, be sure your thigh and shin and your shin and foot are at right angles.

- Lean into your hands to lengthen your back leg as you push the heel down to the mat.

4. **Half downward-facing dog**: Exhale as you step your left leg back to meet the right.

- Push away with your hands, reaching your tailbone back and hinging at the hips until your back is parallel to the floor and makes a right angle with your legs. Engage your quads, pulling the knees up (but not locking them). Raise your hands on the wall slightly if your hamstrings are tight or you feel any twinge in your lower back.

- Keep pressing your tailbone back as you reach the crown of your head toward the wall.

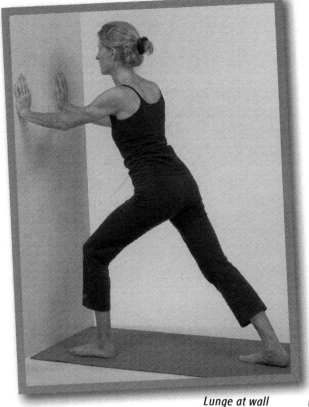

Lunge at wall

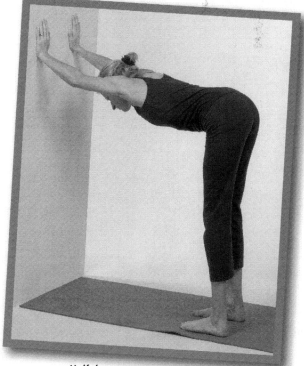

Half dog

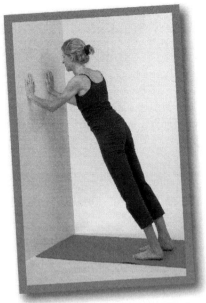

Plank

5. **Plank**: Inhale as you pull your hips and abdomen forward, letting your arms and feet bear the weight as your body straightens.

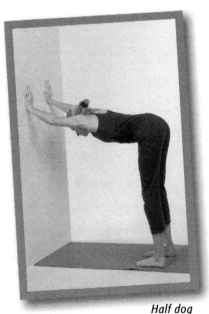

Half dog

6. Exhale back to half downward-facing dog.

7. Inhale as you step the right leg forward into a lunge. Exhale.

8. Inhale as you step the left leg forward and roll up into mountain pose.

9. Inhale into an upward salute. Exhale your arms to your sides and take a resting breath in mountain pose.

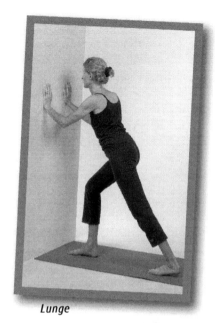

Lunge

10. Repeat Steps 2 through 9 but reach back with the left leg in lunge.

11. Inhale into an upward salute.

12. Exhale your hands down into prayer position over your heart.

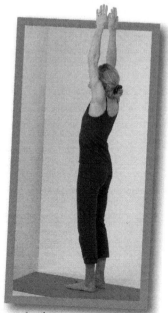

Upward salute

13. Take a resting breath. Feel your heart with the backs of your thumbs. If you stated an intention or affirmation, this is a nice time to repeat it to yourself.

14. Move into the Relaxation that follows.

RELAXATION: GUIDED IMAGERY

Lie in a comfortable position, warmed by blankets and supported by pillows or bolsters as needed. An eye pillow (remove glasses or contact lenses first) may be soothing in this guided imagery exercise.

Take a deep breath in. On the exhale, release tension, negative thoughts, planning, to-do lists.

Imagine that you're on a beach, your favorite beach or one you create for yourself in your mind. With ease, you settle onto the sand.

Feel the sun on your face. It is not a burning sun; it is warm. Remember it from before the warm-ups? Let its warmth penetrate your skin. Feel the heat on your sleeves, your arms and shoulders. Let them all soften into the sand that has shaped itself to the contours of your body, supporting your head, back, legs. Relax into the sand as the sun warms you.

There's a light breeze on this beach. Allow the air to dance on your skin. Smell the sea in the breeze. Listen to the sounds it brings, the waves gently lapping on shore. In and out. Match your breath to the rhythm of the waves. Allow the in breath to bring with it all that is good. Bring that goodness into your being. Exhale out anything that does not nurture you. Let it go out to sea with the outgoing waves. Inhale and feel all that is good permeate through you just as the sun has.

Warm, supported. Nurtured. The sun is shining, the breeze dancing, the waves moving in and out. Rhythmically. Peacefully. Rhythmically. Peacefully.

Lie on this peaceful beach for several more moments.

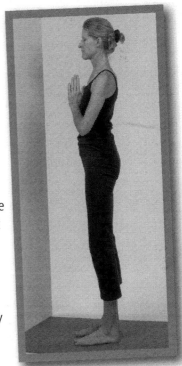

Before opening your eyes, begin to bring your awareness back to the room, to your body, to the moment. Wiggle your fingers and toes in the sand, wrinkle your nose up at the sun. And smile. Know that you can go to this beach, this place of peace at any time. It is yours.

May the warm sun shine upon you. May love surround you. May peace fill you. Namaste.

Namaste

ESPECIALLY BENEFICIAL

- With some movement disorders, our voices can soften. The upward salute increases the space between our ribs where the intercostal muscles are that help us breathe, allowing for more oxygen when we inhale. Good lung capacity can result in stronger voice projection.

- Upward salute and forward bend can loosen the cervical disks and surrounding ligaments of the neck, which can become particularly stiff.

- Weight-bearing on the shoulder muscles in half dog or down dog helps to strengthen the upper body, which can be useful when turning in bed at night.

- Falling can be a concern with the muscle weakness and imbalance that accompany Parkinson's, MS, stroke and other disorders. Weight-bearing on the shoulders aids in building strong bones so we don't break anything if we do stumble.

- The iliopsoas muscle (made up of two connecting muscles) runs from the upper thigh at the head of the femur around to the lower spine. This major muscle can get overly rigid, not only affecting our gait in walking but also tweaking the lower back. Lunges help stretch and release this muscle.

YOGA TO GO: APPLYING IT TO YOUR DAY

- Go outside. Sit or hold onto a railing for balance. Close your eyes and turn your face up toward the sun for a minute or two. Take a deep breath and feel the warmth.

- Watch a sunrise. Notice the changes in color, in the air.

- Watch a sunset. Watch another one a day or two later and note how it's different.

- Take a nap near a sunny window. Rest and restore in the glow.

- Say something kind and warming to yourself.

- Release your spine before bed. Forward bends can be calming to the nervous system. Before turning in at night, sit on the edge of the bed and gently bend forward, hinging at the hips with a straight back (place your hands on your thighs for support). Then let your back curl before slowly rolling back up. This may help with sleep.

- Stretch your spine in the morning. Back extensions (or, arching back) are said to stimulate the nervous system. A soft, easy back extension like in an upward salute might shake off drowsiness in the morning.

- Move into half downward-facing dog (Step 4 of the wall-supported standing variation) at the kitchen sink, the bathroom counter, in the aisle on an airplane for a spine awakener.

- Take yourself to the beach, literally or figuratively, using the beach in your mind's eye from the relaxation. Either way, get to the beach. Often.

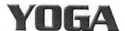
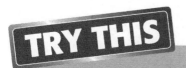

EYE PILLOWS ON HAND

It can be a challenge to soften muscles during Relaxation when fists are involuntarily clenched, or the tremor in one arm won't let it rest. Try this: Place an eye pillow or light sandbag in your palms to help alleviate the tension (even if it's only one hand that needs the weight, it's a nice balance to place one in each palm). In cool temperatures, store the eye pillows on a radiator or heat vent so that they are warm for relaxation time.

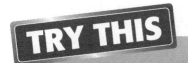

PARTNER UP

Sunday schedules often include family visits. Young children are naturals at yoga and sun salutations can be fun to do together with the kids or grandkids. During the warm-ups, meow and bark during cat and dog stretches. Wag your tails. When greeting the sun, wave, or hold a beach ball between your hands. When bowing to the earth, imagine what's there in the grass beneath your feet. Hiss into cobra. Have some fun.

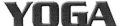
Chapter 5
MONDAY: KNOW IT IS THERE

> **'I like to think that the moon is there even if I am not looking at it,**
> **– Albert Einstein**

A posting to one of my blog entries asked if I experience times when I'm out on errands feeling energized and cruise along and others where I step into the same space dragging and unbalanced.

For many of us, these "on" and "off" times relate to the varying effects of our medications. Factors include time of day, the quality of sleep the night before, what we ate near dosage time, what phase the moon is in. Actually, I made up that last one. But, as I posted in my reply to the blog question, I refer to the "on" and "off" times as waxing and waning. My true energy, I believe, is there whether I can see it or not.

A similar energy exists with yoga, even when we're not looking. Yoga's mind/body connection is there, it's waiting for us to notice.

ASANA PRACTICE

The moon series, or *chandra namaskar*, is cooling. The flow is a good way to end the day. Or, move through the series if you're trying not to overheat, as controlling our body temperature can be a challenge with movement disorders. This flow can also be

calming at times when tone or tremor is particularly active.

Like the sun salutation, moon poses invite opposing forces to work while maintaining a balanced center. This asana flow focuses on strengthening and stretching the muscles that allow the legs to kick forward and back and turn in and out – the hip flexors and extenders as well as the adductors and abductors that move the legs sideways.

The poses in this series resemble the moon as it moves through its phases. But know, too, that they also work the legs. To avoid fatigue, try only the first three steps for a few weeks. When you feel comfortable proceeding through the series, pause at any time, particularly between steps, to take a resting breath.

There are numerous variations on the moon series. In each, the flow reaches to the sky while solidly grounded. Throughout the poses, feel your feet and knees press onto the mat or sitting bones onto the chair. At the same time, feel the reach as a lift from the tailbone up through the heart and out the crown of the head.

As the moon spreads an even glow, reflecting the light of the sun, this flow can create a calming way to shine from within.

Coming to Stillness

Find a comfortable, straight-backed position on a cushion, on the mat or on a chair, with your palms resting on your knees or with your hands on a pillow in your lap.

Inhale deeply.

On the next exhale, breathe out anything that is not calming – your to-do list, a mental replay of an argument, pain, the driver who cut you off – exhale it all. Picture your outgoing breath as hot, smoggy, heavy, like the hazy sun on a sweltering day.

As you inhale, image a pristine lake reflecting the moonrise. Breathe in the cool, crisp, clean night air.

Follow this for two more breaths, relaxing in the image of the white glow on deep, clear water.

Warm-ups

Please refer to Chapter 3 for the warm-up exercises to do before practicing the following flow. Work through all of Set A and poses 4 and 5 from Set B.

Poses

MOON SERIES

Seated Variation

Need: Sticky mat
Straight-backed chair
Blocks, books, or firm blanket (optional)

Difficulty: Any level can try this flow.

Spread your mat and place the chair on a short end, seat facing the mat. Be sure all four legs of the chair are on the mat to prevent slipping. Ideally, spread the mat where there's a wall arm's length away. This could help if you need to reach out for balance.

1. Sit in seated mountain pose.

2. **Crescent moon**: Inhale and let the breath lead you as you slowly raise both arms to the sky. Clasp fingers, with index fingers pointing up in temple position.

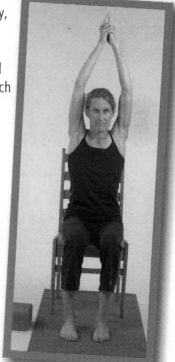

Moon series on a chair:
crescent moon

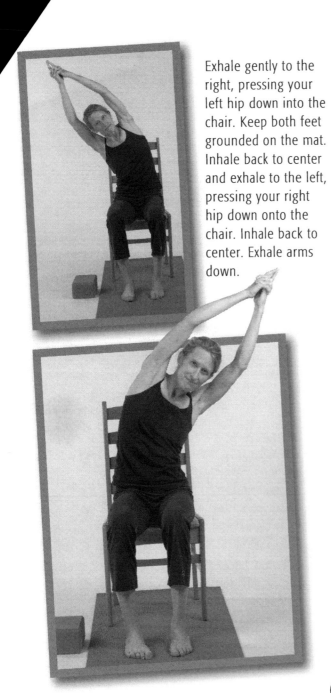

Exhale gently to the right, pressing your left hip down into the chair. Keep both feet grounded on the mat. Inhale back to center and exhale to the left, pressing your right hip down onto the chair. Inhale back to center. Exhale arms down.

3. **Goddess**: Step your feet about shoulder-width apart. Inhale and raise your arms to a T position, then on an exhale, bend your elbows, fingers pointing up and palms facing each other. If this feels comfortable, remain in the pose for an extra breath or two. Release your arms. Shake out your arms and take a resting breath.

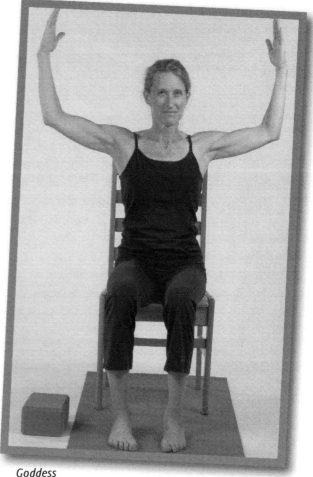

Goddess

4. **Seated forward bend with twist**: With a straight back, exhale and hinge forward placing your hands on the floor or on a block. Center your right hand on the block. On an inhale, sweep your left arm up to the sky. If it is comfortable, look up at your fingertips. Exhale and release your arm down and repeat with your right arm.

- Optional: If it is not comfortable for you to reach your arm up, place your right hand on your knee and look over your right shoulder. Repeat for the left side.

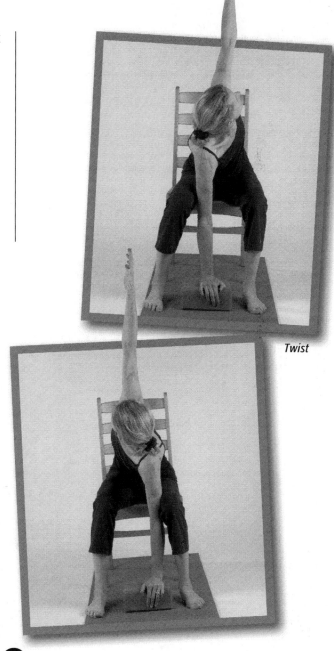

Twist

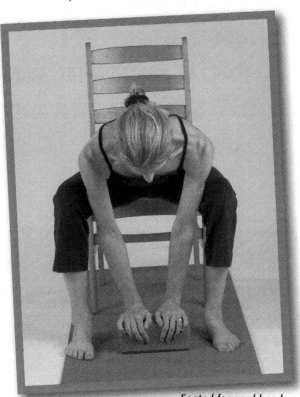

Seated forward bend

5. **Seated hamstring stretch**: Come back into seated mountain pose at the edge of your chair. Stretch your right leg straight in front of you, foot flexed, your left leg bent with knee and ankle at 90 degree angles. Place your hands on the chair for support as you exhale and hinge forward from the hips. Feel that your spine is straight, not rounded. If your hamstrings feel especially tight, sit up some. Release back to mountain and switch legs.

   • Optional: If your feet don't reach the floor to form a comfortable right angle at the ankle, place your feet on blocks, a phone book or books, or a firm, folded blanket.

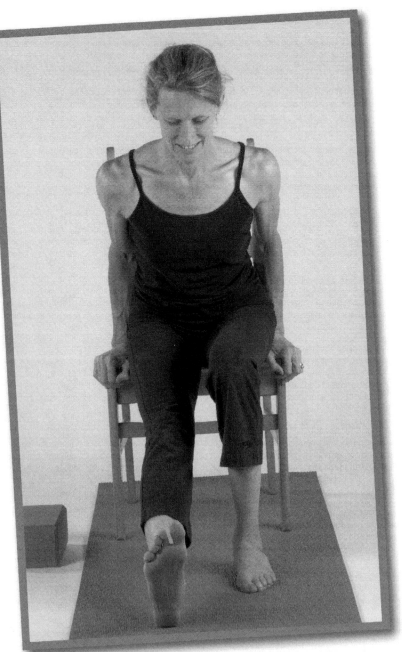

Seated hamstring stretch

6. **Goddess**: Reposition yourself on the chair so you are facing forward. Repeat Step 3.

7. **Crescent Moon**: Repeat Step 2.

8. Take a resting breath. Prepare for the Relaxation that follows.

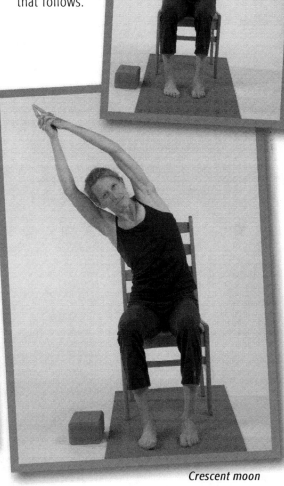

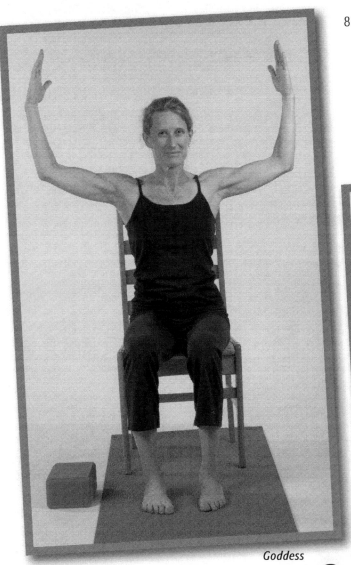

Goddess

Crescent moon

MOON SERIES

Supported Standing Variation

Need: Sticky mat
Straight-backed chair
Block

Difficulty: This can be a challenging flow if you have balance concerns or are new to stretching. Try the seated variation first.

Spread your mat and place the chair on a short end of it, the seat facing the mat. Be sure all four legs of the chair are on the mat to prevent slipping. Ideally, spread the mat where there's a wall arm's length away. This could help if you need to reach out for balance.

If you're fearful of falling, please use the seated variation.

1. Stand in mountain pose to the left of the seat of the chair, about six inches away from it.

2. **Crescent moon**: Inhale and let the breath lead you as you slowly raise both arms to the sky. Clasp fingers, with index fingers pointing up in temple position. Notice if your elbows are straight but not locked. Exhale your upper body gently to the right, allowing your left hip to glide slightly left, but keeping weight even on both feet. Inhale back to center and exhale to the left, allowing your right hip to glide slightly right, weight even on both feet. Inhale back to center. Exhale arms down.

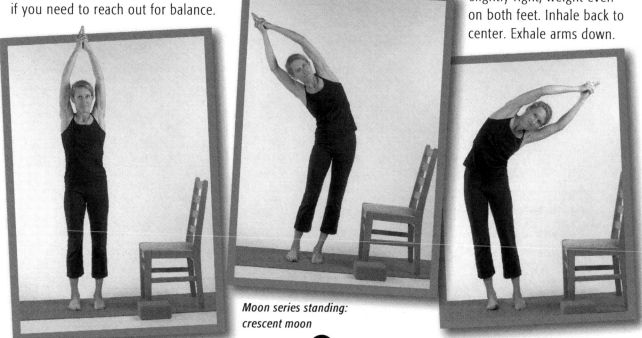

Moon series standing: crescent moon

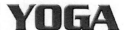
3. **Goddess**: Step your feet about shoulder-width apart, toes pointing outward, about 30 degrees. Bend your knees slightly. (Caution: Be certain that the bent knee is not extending past the ankle; there should be a right angle at the ankle, the knee directly over it. You should be able to see your big toes.) Raise arms to a T position, then bend elbows, fingers pointing up and palms facing each other. If this feels comfortable, remain in the pose for an extra breath or two.

- Try to keep your torso straight, as though a line runs from your nose to your navel to the center point on the mat between your feet.
- Feel the contact with the ground through your feet as you reach through your fingertips and crown of your head, keeping your shoulders relaxed.

4. With an inhale, straighten your legs and release your arms to your waist.

5. **Wide-angle forward bend**: Lengthen up on an inhale. With the exhale, leading with your heart, hinge forward at the hips and place your hands on the floor or on a block. Bend your knees if you feel any strain in your lower back or hamstrings.

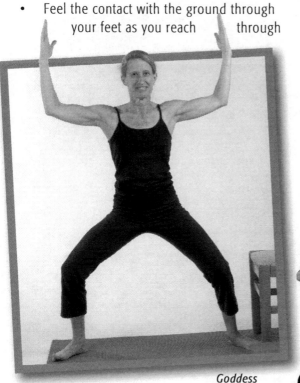

Goddess

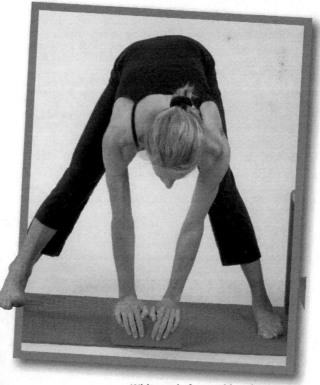

Wide-angle forward bend

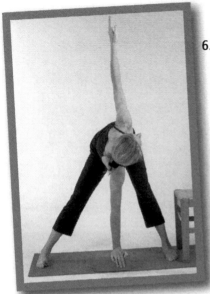

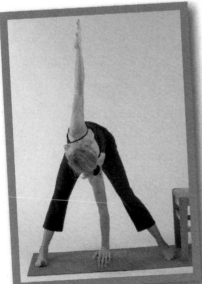

Twist

6. **Twist**: Center your right hand on the block. On an inhale, sweep your left arm up to the sky. If it is comfortable, look up at your fingertips. On an exhale, release your arm down and repeat with your right arm.

7. Come back to center, inhaling as you press into your feet and roll back up to standing.

8. **Standing Head to Knee**: Stand and pivot your feet to face the chair. Your right foot is now behind you, your left foot forward. Keeping your legs straight, hinge forward at the hips. Place your hands on the chair and, if possible, bow your head toward your left knee. If your hamstrings feel especially tight, bow your head to the chair seat rather than your knee.

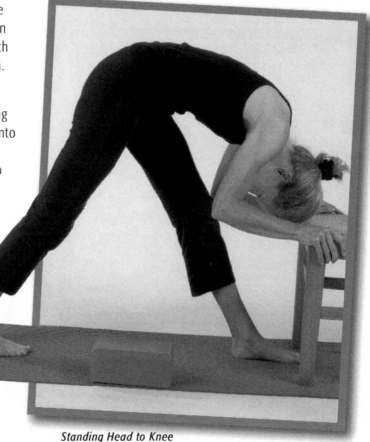

Standing Head to Knee

9. **Kneeling Warrior**: From standing head to knee, use the chair to support your upper body with your hands as you drop to your right knee, which is slightly behind your hip. Bend the left at 90 degrees. (Caution: Be certain that the bent knee is not extending past the ankle; there should be a right angle at the ankle, the knee stacked directly over it. You should be able to see the big toe of your left foot.) Use one or both hands on the chair for balance. If you feel balanced, supported by your grounded left foot, leave your left hand on the chair with a light touch and raise your right fingertips to the sky. Breathe into the stretch, allowing your hips to come slightly forward.

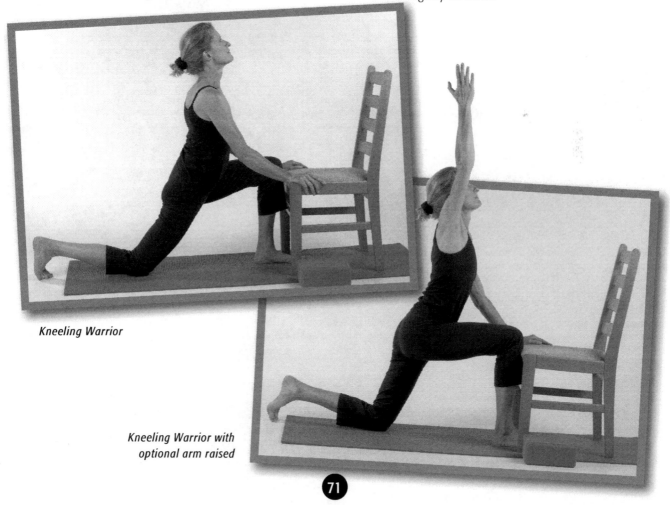

Kneeling Warrior

Kneeling Warrior with optional arm raised

10. **Switch**: Bring your left knee to the mat then back and your right leg forward, the right foot on the mat and the knee at 90 degrees. If you feel balanced, supported by your grounded right foot and right hand, raise your left fingertips to the sky. Breathe into the stretch in your left thigh's quad and psoas muscles.

11. **Standing Head to Knee**: With your hands on the chair for support, straighten both legs and bow forward as in Step 8.

12. **Wide-angle forward bend**: Stand and pivot your feet to the left so you are sideways on the mat. Repeat Step 5, facing the opposite way.

Standing Head to Knee

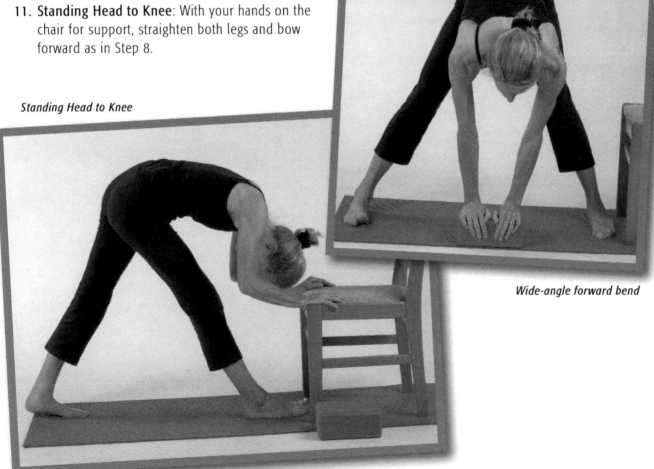

Wide-angle forward bend

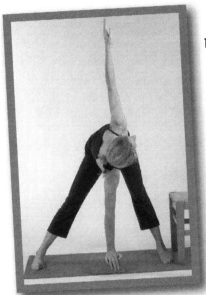

13. Twist: Repeat Step 6. Inhale to standing.

Twist

14. Goddess: Repeat Step 3.

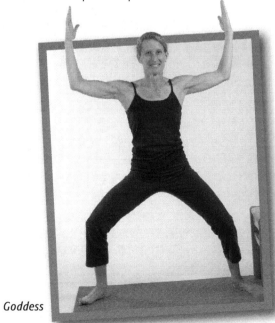

Goddess

15. Crescent Moon: Repeat Step 2.

16. Take a resting breath. Prepare for the Relaxation that follows.

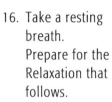

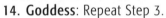

Crescent moon

...N: GUIDED IMAGERY

Lie or sit, perhaps with legs up on a facing chair, in a comfortable position, warmed by blankets and supported by pillows or bolsters as needed. Again, an eye pillow (remove glasses or contact lenses first) may be soothing in this guided imagery exercise.

Inhale, then exhale fully. Take a deep breath in to the count of four. Pause to the count of four. Exhale completely. Repeat this one more time before returning to your natural breath. Feel your back supported by the floor or chair back, the back of your shoulders, your upper back, your sacrum and hips.

Recall the moonlight you brought to mind during Coming to Stillness. It's a pure, clean light reflecting off the lake. Let that light enter through the crown of your head, illuminating cells with its cool, healing presence. Watch the light as it moves down into the neck and shoulders, shining into dark corners. Follow the clean, white path it makes as it lights the spine, organs, hips and legs down through the feet and into each toe.

Allow the moonlight reflection to return to the water, breathing in the cool, clear air off the lake. Rest for a few more minutes, supported, cleansed, healing.

Before opening your eyes, begin to bring your awareness back to the room, to your body, to the moment. Wiggle your fingers and toes, wrinkle your

nose. And smile. Know that the pure healing light of the moon is always there, even if you can't see it.

May you be supported, as the night sky holds the moon, allowing you to shine through every phase that is you. Namaste.

ESPECIALLY BENEFICIAL

- Strong, flexible hip/groin muscles support us, help us walk. And dance.

- Stroke recovery can still leave us walking with a limp. Strengthening the legs helps both legs carry the load.

- The uneven gait that comes with a stroke or with movement disorders such as Parkinson's can affect the lower back. Keeping our hamstrings from getting too tight helps take some stress off the lumbar and sacral joints of the back and hips.

- Weight-bearing on the legs in goddess pose can help maintain strong pelvic bones, which can can be beneficial against developing osteoporosis.

- In head to knee, the heart is higher than the brain, creating an inversion of blood flow, which can help create a sense of calm, even sleepiness. Will it cure the insomnia related

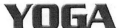
to movement disorders or side effects of medication? No, but it can help.

YOGA TO GO: APPLYING IT TO YOUR DAY

- Look at the moon tonight. How much of it can you see? Is it waxing or waning?

- Check a lunar calendar to see what phases the moon will go through over the next two weeks. Notice what changes you go through in the same timeframe.

- Notice the night air. Breathe it in. Is it heavier or lighter than it was during the day?

- Make note of something that, like yoga or the moon, is always there for you. Your breath. Your heartbeat. The chance to say something kind to yourself.

- Dance. In the shower, in the kitchen, with someone you love. A study by a team of researchers at Washington University School of Medicine in St. Louis found that the tango helps people with Parkinson's with balance and mobility.

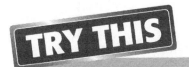

WAKE-UP YOGA

A refreshing way to begin the day is with some yoga before getting out of bed. Try this: Lie on your back and take a deep breath in and out. Focus on the air moving from the tip of your nose down into your expanding ribs. Feel your belly rise and then fall with your outgoing breath. Take another inhale and on an exhale, pull one knee to your chest. On the next exhale, pull the other knee up, too. Wrap your arms around your shins, or knees, or wherever they reach, and hug your legs close, without lifting your head. Release, stretch long and take one more full, deep breath. On the exhale: smile. Sometimes this is the only yoga that will fit into the day. Or, maybe you'll greet each day this way. I do.

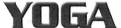
Chapter 6
TUESDAY: TWIST IT

'And the stars look very
different today,
'Space Oddity, – David Bowie

Early in the dating phase of our relationship, my husband and I were out on a walk. We met up with a man he knew from graduate school. On introducing me, my husband said, "This is" – *pause* – "this is my, um, friend."

We laugh about it now, my "umfriend" label. No matter how any of us try not to label ourselves or others, it's often how we identify ourselves. We're parents, children, dentists, cyclists, patients. Yoga reminds us that there's more than being the umfriend, the neighbor, the label. It turns us inward to self-reflect, to look at not only what we do but at who we are.

ASANA PRACTICE

Twists encourage vertebrae to move, rotate. This turning of the torso also gives organs a healthy squeeze and can be helpful in relieving constipation.

As we wring out the muscles along the spine, we release tension caught there. In turn, the motion can soothe tension caught elsewhere: in our minds. This spiraling motion also reminds us that we begin and return to the starting point: ourselves.

In a twist, we can reflect and take a moment to recoil before springing back into the action of daily living. But, remember to focus on what's going on in your body. Notice when you're moving into twists that you allow your hips to shift with the motion. Locking them in place can strain the ligaments in the sacrum where the tailbone attaches to the pelvis. And allow yourself to move to where your body allows, to where you feel it is today, not to where you think it should be.

Coming to Stillness

Sit in a comfortable, straight-backed position on a chair, with your palms resting on your knees or with your hands on a pillow in your lap.

Inhale fully. Feel the air enter, from the tip of the nose down the back of your throat. Notice if breath comes in at the top or bottom of the nasal passage. Is the air warm or cool? Allow this full breath to fill to the base of your lungs.

Exhale deeply, squeezing the air out fully. Notice if the breath exits at the top or bottom of the nasal passage. Is it warm or cool?

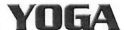

Rub your palms together briskly to warm them. Once warmed, place your cupped palms gently over your closed eyes. Feel the heat through your eyelids. Let your hands block out light, tension, to-do lists. Breathe at your regular rate for several cycles of breath before removing your hands from your eyes.

Warm-ups

Please refer to Chapter 3 for the warm-up exercises to do before practicing the following flow. Work through all of Set A and poses 2 and 7 (if you're comfortable standing) from Set B.

Poses

If you have any concern about falling from the chair in these poses, place your chair beside a wall. Reach out to the wall for balance at any time.

Twists can alleviate back pain. At times, twists aggravate back pain, particularly when muscles are in spasm. Should you experience discomfort or pain in your back during a twist, come out of the pose.

TWIST

Seated Twist

> *Need: Straight-backed chair*
> *Sticky mat*

Difficulty: Any level can try this pose.

This asana eases up from the base to the top of the spine.

1. Sit sideways on the chair, feet on the floor with ankles at a 90-degree angle (add a blanket or cushion beneath your feet if your legs aren't long enough for your feet to rest this way).

2. Place both hands on the back of the chair, very lightly gripping it.

3. Inhaling, lengthen your spine by pressing up through the crown of your head and down with your sitting bones onto the chair.

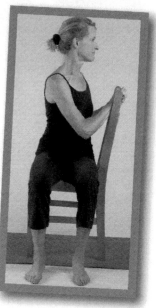

Seated twist

4. Exhaling, twist at your base, turning toward the back of the chair. Allow the tailbone to turn and then your hips. Keep your chin in line with your sternum, or breastbone.

5. Inhaling, pause and lengthen your spine.

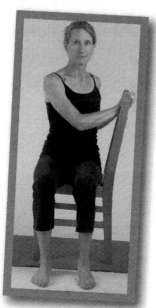

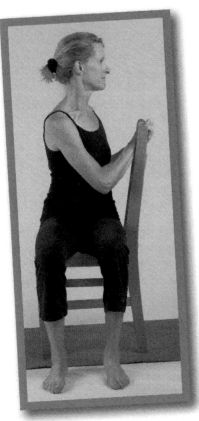

6. Exhaling, twist at your middle, turning your rib cage toward the back of the chair. With a light touch, you can use your arms to assist in the twist.

7. Inhaling, lengthen your spine.

8. Exhaling, twist at your shoulders.

9. Inhaling, lengthen your spine.

10. Exhaling, let your chin turn toward the back of the chair and gaze over your shoulder.

11. To come out of the twist, release your head and then hands and slowly uncoil.

12. Take a resting breath before sitting sideways in the other direction on the chair, following the steps to twist on that side.

13. Take a resting breath before moving to the next asana.

TWIST

Standing Twist at Wall
> *Need: Straight-backed, armless chair*

Difficulty: Anyone who can stand comfortably can try this pose.

This pose can help with fatigue.

1. Position your chair with the back against a wall. Stand with your right shoulder touching the wall and step your right leg onto the chair. Place a block or folded towel under your foot if you need to so that your thigh is parallel with the floor, your hip and knee at right angles.

2. Place your palms on the wall.

3. Inhale and press down through both feet, extending up through the crown of your head.

4. Exhale and turn toward the wall, using your hands for support.

5. Stay in the twist for several seconds, working up to a minute over time.

6. Stepping your right foot back down, take a moment to shake out both arms and legs.

7. Stand on the other side of the chair with your left shoulder touching the wall and repeat on the left side.

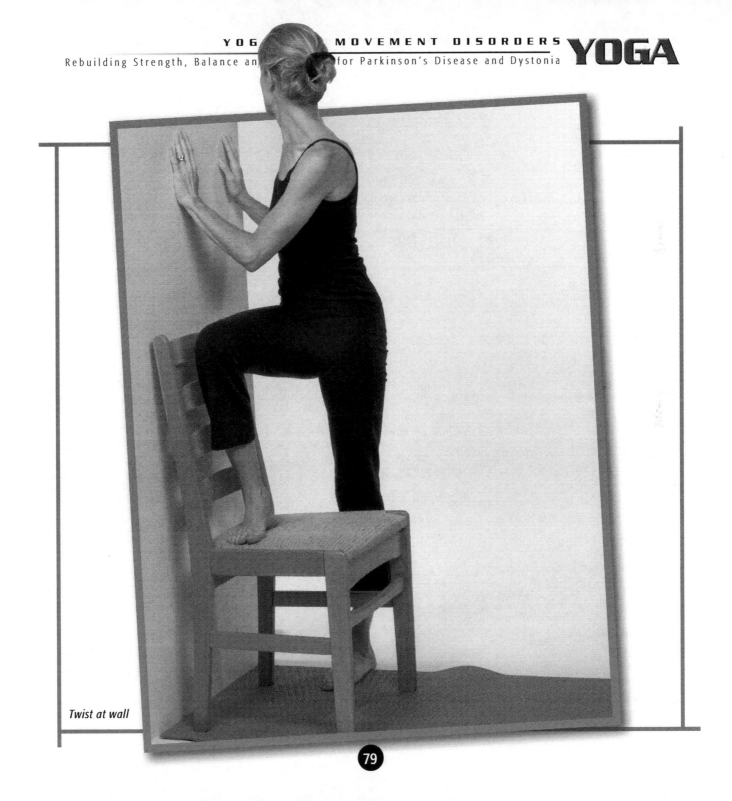

Twist at wall

TWIST

Cross-legged Twist

Need: Mat
Blanket or cushion or bolster
Blocks (optional)

Difficulty: Anyone who doesn't have difficulty getting to the floor comfortably can try this pose.

This pose helps release the lower back.

1. Sit cross-legged on the mat. Use a folded blanket or cushion or bolster to raise your sitting bones so your back is straight and your hips are positioned slightly forward. The higher you are seated, the easier it is to sit with a straight back. If your back is rounded, even on the bolster, skip this asana and prepare for the Relaxation that follows.

2. Place cushions or blocks under your knees for support, particularly if your groin muscles are tight.

3. Place your right hand on your left knee.

4. Inhale as you lengthen up and exhale as you twist from the abdomen to the left.

5. Lighten the pressure into your right sitting bone as you twist, keeping the hip free to follow the movement.

6. Inhale as you lengthen up and exhale as you continue the twist from the ribs and, with the next two rounds of breath, from the shoulders and head.

7. Untwist and repeat on the left side.

8. Untwist and take a resting breath.

9. Prepare for the Relaxation that follows. Use a folded blanket for a pillow, another blanket over you for warmth.

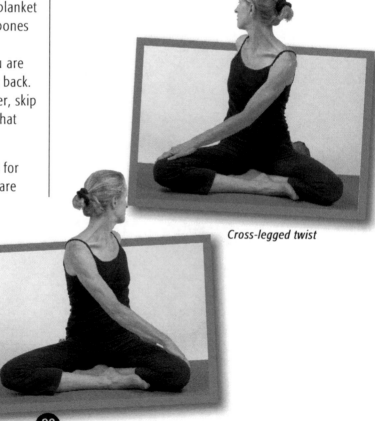

Cross-legged twist

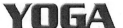

TWIST

Knees-down Twist

Need: Sticky mat

Difficulty: Anyone who doesn't have difficulty getting to the floor comfortably can try this pose.

This pose helps release the lower back.

1. Lie on the mat on your back, knees bent and feet flat on the mat about hip width apart. Take a cycle or two of breath to allow your body to settle onto the floor, feeling how it supports your hips and shoulders.

2. On an inhale, reach your arms out into a T position. If this is uncomfortable or triggers any tremor, try reaching out into a T position with bent elbows. Allow your forearms to rest on the mat on either side of your head, palms facing up.

3. With the back of your head on the mat, gaze upward and allow your knees to drop down to one side, back to center, and then to the other side, back and forth like windshield wipers.

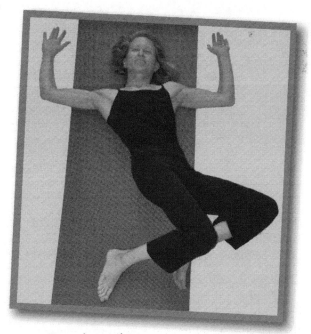

Knees-down twist

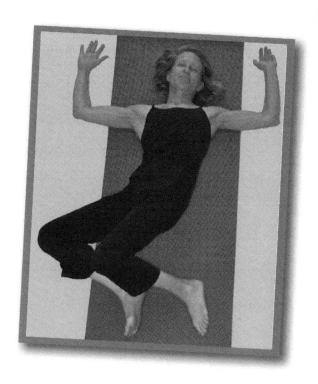

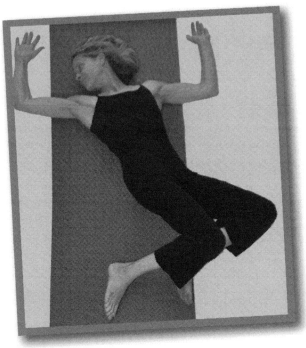

4. After several sweeps from side to side, the next time your knees move to the right, allow them to remain there for a cycle or two of breath. Don't strain to press your knees to the floor. Simply allow them to rest there. Bring your attention to keeping the back of your left shoulder on the mat. If it is comfortable on your neck, turn your head to gaze over your left fingertips or elbow.

5. Bring your head back to center and knees back to center. Allow your knees to flop from side to side several more times. The next time your knees move to the left, allow them to remain there for a cycle or two of breath and turn your head to gaze over your right fingertips or elbow.

6. Bring your head back to center and prepare for the Relaxation that follows. Use a folded blanket for a pillow, another blanket over you for warmth.

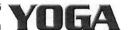
RELAXATION: GUIDED IMAGERY

Lie in a comfortable position, warmed by blankets and supported by pillows or bolsters as needed. Again, an eye pillow (remove glasses or contact lenses first) may be soothing in this guided imagery exercise.

Inhale deeply and release the breath with an audible sigh. Prepare to go to a favorite place – a cabin in the woods, your childhood home – a place that's warm and comfortable and safe.

Drive there in a sporty car or ride on horseback or on the wings of a bird. When you get there, find a spot to lie down and relax. Settle in.

What colors are there in your favorite place?

What do you hear there? Birdsong? Laughter?

Can you smell the ocean? Or new-mown grass?

What is you favorite treat there? Can you taste it?

What do your fingers reach out and touch? Sand? The velvet fur of a dog's ear?

For several minutes, relax into this safe, warm, comfortable place with all your senses.

Before opening your eyes, begin to bring your awareness back to the room, to your body, to the moment. Wiggle your fingers and toes, wrinkle your nose. Take a deep breath in – maybe you can still smell the scents of your favorite place. Exhale knowing you can go back to this place anytime, not to do anything there but to safely be who you are.

May you be at peace. Namaste.

ESPECIALLY BENEFICIAL

- Our trunk muscles around the waist and hips get tight with various movement disorders. Twists help release the grip.

- With an uneven gait, particularly if a stroke has affected the nerves on one side of the body, the lower back can get strained. Twists help reset the vertebrae and muscle fibers to relieve that strain.

- If you drive, being able to turn to look behind you is safer than relying solely on the rearview mirror.

- Parkinson's can cause a stoop when standing and the imbalance in muscle strength from a stroke or MS affects how straight we stand. Twists can help our posture by releasing tightness in the back and by strengthening the shoulders and arms as they assist in the movement.

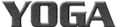
YOGA TO GO: APPLYING IT TO YOUR DAY

- Webster's defines *layoff* as a period of inactivity or idleness. Each day, lay off something on your to-do list. Breathe and be for those few moments.

- Typically, when someone asks us what we do, we respond by switching to the verb form of *be*. I *am* a vet, gardener, student. The next time, answer using the verb *do*. Notice if that changes how you identify who you are.

- If you sit for long periods – at a desk, in the car – and your back feels tight, twist it. Airplanes are an especially good place to twist. Restaurants can be, too.

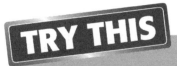

TAP DANCE

When all the concentration you can muster still doesn't get some body part to move, try this: tap. Specifically, lightly touch the part you want to move with the tips of your fingers. For example, if you're turning in bed from your side to your stomach, tap on the back of the hip. It doesn't work every time, but often it does. Tapping helps the brain make the connection to the muscles that internal chemistry isn't doing.

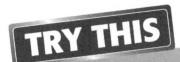

FACE IT

Tension often builds up in the neck and shoulders. Another common area where tension and rigidity hide is in our face. Take a few minutes to put on a happy face, or a surprised face, or a dismayed face. Make a face. Squeeze your brows and lips into an eew, yuck face or puff your cheeks into a clown face. Go ahead and smile.

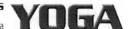

Chapter 7
WEDNESDAY: FOLLOW YOUR BREATH

'Everything is all right if I just breathe,
— **Michelle Branch**

Despite the stickers on the glass, birds still fly across my back deck into the sliding doors. A female grosbeak hit hard one summer day. She landed belly up, her chest rising and falling in quick breaths.

I ached to scoop her up in a towel and take her to the nearby sanctuary for injured wild birds. I knew not to interfere, though. Not yet. Give it a little time. Besides her breathing, all that moved were her eyes, and I sensed she saw me looking at her. It was an unnatural sight, her underside exposed, legs sprawled. I felt like I'd caught a glimpse of someone behind a hospital curtain, pale and mouth agape.

Busying myself in the kitchen, I put dishes away as though my doing an everyday task would help the bird get back to normal. I checked her again. She'd righted herself, but was crooked and quite still but for her breathing. I found another chore to do before glancing out at her again. Still crooked. Still breathing. I opened mail, made a sandwich. Still on the deck, but still breathing. Thinking it might be time to wrap her in the towel, I looked out again. She was gone.

The stunned bird hadn't sung out. She didn't stretch a wing. Instinctually, she simply breathed. Wherever our yoga journeys take us – to sun salutations atop a mountain peak or restorative poses in the comfort of our own rooms – we must breathe. It centers us, brings healing. Breathe and we can soar.

ASANA PRACTICE

Beyond asana practice, there is also breathing practice or pranayama. *Prana* means breath and includes the life energy that fills us as we breathe. *Pranayama* translates as regulating the breath, or, loosely, breathing exercises.

Notice your breathing when someone cuts you off in traffic. It becomes short, shallow, carrying little oxygen and signaling stress to the rest of the body. Notice your breathing when you're enjoying a good book. It is rhythmic, deep. It lets the body know there's no need for alarm. By focusing on our breath, we can bring our awareness to what's going on in our bodies as well as our minds, regulating and balancing the energy within both.

Coming to Stillness

Breathing through the mouth can cause restlessness. Inhaling through the mouth can introduce air into the stomach. This can result in discomfort and burping. Whenever possible, allow air to flow through the nose on inhales and exhales.

Find a comfortable, straight-backed position on a cushion, on the mat or on a chair, with your palms resting on your knees. Take three regular breaths.

On the next inhalation, place your hands on your belly. Breathe in and let your belly press into your palms. Exhale and feel the belly contract.

The diaphragm, which spans the area beneath the lungs, is our main muscle for respiration. On the inhale, it lengthens, flattens.

"Belly" breathing is when we allow the expansion to press down, expanding the belly area wider. This first step begins to fill the lungs from the bottom up.

Next, place your hands on your rib cage. Allow the inhale to expand the belly and, taking in a bit more air, let it expand your ribs. This step fills the bottom and the middle of the lungs. Exhale, letting your ribs return to neutral.

Bring your fingertips to your upper chest, just beneath your collarbone. Breathe in and expand your belly, your ribs, and then your upper chest. Feel your fingertips rise with the inhale. Exhale. Pushing the air out, feel your upper chest lower, your rib cage drop, your belly contract. This third step completes the exercise, breathing into the bottom, middle, and top of the lungs.

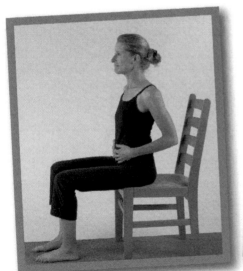
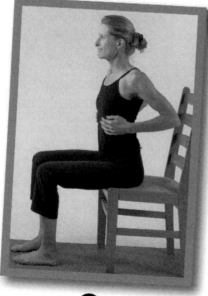
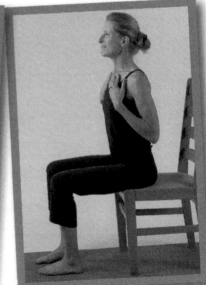

86 *Three-part breath*

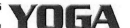
Breathe this way for one more cycle of breath, and imagine inhaling good, nurturing energy and exhaling out anything that is stale or negative.

Warm-ups

Please refer to Chapter 3 for the warm-up exercises to do before practicing the following breathing exercises. Work through all of Set A.

Poses

Breath control can be energizing or calming, depending on the pattern of breathing. By changing our breathing pattern, we can alter that state and the stresses it has on our bodies.

BREATH EXERCISES

Bee Breath or Humming Breath
Need: Straight-backed chair

Difficulty: Anyone can try this exercise.

This breathing exercise can be helpful for anxiety. For added centering, try using earplugs and/or closing your eyes.

1. Sit comfortably on your sitting bones. Lengthen your spine by pressing your sitting bones down onto the chair as you reach up through the crown of your head.

2. Inhale fully through your nose.

3. With mouth closed, jaw relaxed, make a humming sound as you exhale. Notice if the vibration is in the roof of your mouth and cheekbones.

4. Breathe this way for three more cycles of breath.

5. Inhale again through your nose.

6. Press your back teeth together gently and make a humming sound as you exhale. Notice if the vibration moves to your sinuses and vertebrae in your neck.

BREATH EXERCISES

Lion's Breath
Need: Straight-backed chair

Difficulty: Anyone can try this exercise.

This is a calming breathing exercise.

1. Sit comfortably on your sitting bones. Lengthen your spine by pressing your sitting bones down onto the chair as you reach up through the crown of your head.

2. Place your hands on your knees, fingers curled like claws.

3. Let your mouth open.

4. As you inhale, tilt your head back slightly, opening your mouth wider.

5. Hinge forward at the hips, sticking your tongue out and exhaling from your throat with an audible *haaa*.

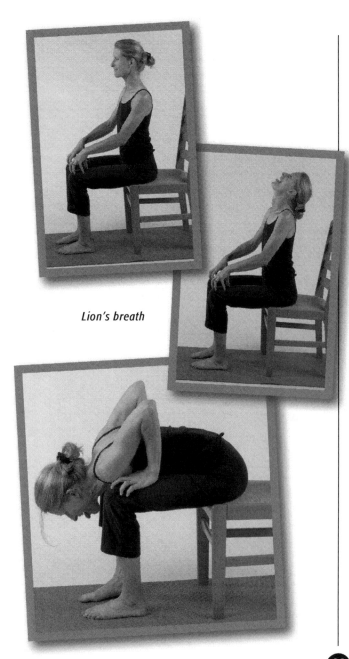

Lion's breath

6. Close your mouth and on an inhale, straighten back up to a seated position.

7. Relax your hands palms-down on your lap and take a resting breath.

8. Repeat steps 2 through 7 two more times, imagining that you are spilling any anger, frustration, or negative thoughts into the earth through your open mouth as you exhale.

BREATH EXERCISES

Counting Breath

Need: Straight-backed chair

Difficulty: Anyone can try this exercise.

This exercise helps focus the mind and settle thoughts. It can be useful before meditation or sleep.

1. Sit comfortably on your sitting bones. Lengthen your spine by pressing your sitting bones down onto the chair as you reach up through the crown of your head.

2. Inhale halfway to the count of four.

3. Pause your breath to the count of four.

4. Inhale the rest of your breath to the count of four.

5. Pause to the count of four.

6. Slowly exhale completely.

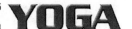
7. Repeat several more times, noticing your belly expand and contract with the inhales and exhales.

8. Prepare for the Relaxation that follows.

RELAXATION: GUIDED IMAGERY

Lie with props as needed under your head and neck, knees, with your back comfortable. Let the blankets and props fully support you.

Breathe regularly and listen to the sounds around you. A car driving down the street, perhaps, or a fan running. Next, listen to the sound of your breath. How quiet can you make it?

Follow that sound inside as your breath expands your belly and ribs. Do you hear anything in your body? An ache, a twinge? Send your breath to any spaces needing expanding or calming.

Recall the good, nurturing energy you started with during Coming to Stillness. Bring that same energy in on the next inhale and let it spread from your forehead down your neck and shoulders. Allow it to permeate your chest, each arm and across your belly and lower back. Feel it releasing your legs and feet. Let it settle into you for a few minutes longer. All you need to do is breathe.

As you begin to bring your awareness back to the room, to your body, take a deep breath in and exhale it with an audible *ahh*. Wiggle your fingers and toes, wrinkle your nose. Pull one knee up to your chest and then the other. Give yourself a hug and rock slightly from side to side. Notice your regular breathing. Is it full? Is it any different than at the beginning of today's practice?

Shanti, shanti: Peace. Namaste.

ESPECIALLY BENEFICIAL

- The rigidity and involuntary muscle contractions that come with Parkinson's and other movement disorders don't always respond to stretching. In fact, stretches can cause more tightening by triggering muscles into further contraction. Breathing can calm these muscles enough to encourage them to let go of their grip.

- Breathing deeply helps increase circulation.

- Deepening your breath can clear your mind.

- Quieting breaths can also prepare us for sleep, which is especially useful with restlessness, a side effect that often accompanies medications for movement disorders.

- Depression is another symptom of disease or side effect of medications. The release of tension and lowering of stress hormones that result from deep breathing exercises can help alleviate the symptoms of mild depression.

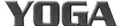
YOGA TO GO: APPLYING IT TO YOUR DAY

- Take note of your breathing pattern at least once a day. Is it shallow or deep, quick or slow?

- Next time you're waiting at the doctor's office, rather than leaf through a magazine, spend a few minutes becoming aware of your breath. Try to deepen your inhales and exhales, filling the belly and rib cage.

- Use the few moments at a red light to take a few full breaths.

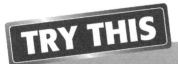

A FOOTBALL TRICK

During breathing exercises, or simply during the Coming to Stillness part of practice, if it's difficult to get air through the nose, as can happen especially with stroke, try this. Use the nasal strips that professional football players wear. The adhesive strips open up the airway for fuller breaths (which means more oxygen in the blood, which means more energy). The strips can be found at most drugstores and are easy to adhere. They even come in clear (and glasses can be worn over them).

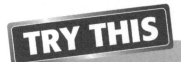

COUNTDOWN

By changing the count in Counting Breath, we can change how we feel between calm and energized. For added relaxation, try the Counting Breath with even inhales and exhales. After a few cycles, keep the length of the inhales the same but increase the length of your exhales by two or more counts. When needing more energy, try the Counting Breath with even inhales and exhales. After a few cycles, keep the length of the exhales the same and increase the length of the inhales by two or more counts.

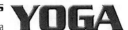
Chapter 8
THURSDAY: STAY STRONG

*'I do believe I'm feeling
stronger every day,
'Feelin' Stronger Every Day,* – Chicago

At the end of class one morning, one student rose from relaxation surprised that she'd moved through the asana practice without her cane. She grinned and glanced around for it. When she realized it was still in the car, she laughed. Other students in class smiled with her.

Still beaming at the unknown strength that had walked in with her, she did express that she felt a bit tired. Everyone volunteered to go out and get the cane for her. The first to spring up was the seventy-five-year-old woman with lupus. What she did, however, was hold out her arm like a human cane. Together, they stepped out the door.

Whatever hidden strength flowed through the two of them, the power of caring and community glowed in their wake.

ASANA PRACTICE

Virabhadrasana, or warrior pose, builds strength and stamina in the face of battles, the everyday challenges as well as the life-changing ones. There are three warrior poses. In the first two, the reach is in opposite directions. The back arm and leg

represent the past and the front limbs symbolize the future. While our hands and feet are reaching for both what was and what will be, our minds and bodies remain centered in the present moment. It's helpful to keep this in mind while in the poses, noticing if your body is leaning forward or back rather than balanced in the middle.

Coming to Stillness

Find a comfortable seated position on your chair or on a cushion on the mat. Press your sitting bones down as you lengthen up through the crown of your head. Inhale deeply through your nose, pause, and exhale.

On the next deep breath in, pause for a moment when your inhale is complete. Exhale to the count of four. Allow the inhale to flow naturally, pausing again before counting the exhale. Repeat this for another cycle or two of breath.

Return to your regular breath but notice if you're feeling anything different in any part of your body. When an anxious moment causes a shortness of breath, this exercise can be useful. Rather than struggling to get air, we can bring our awareness to the exhale and let the inhale simply happen.

Warm-ups

Please refer to Chapter 3 for the warm-up exercises to do before practicing the following asana flow. Work through all of Set A and 1, 4, and 6 from Set B.

STRENGTH POSES

Seated Warrior Flow

Need: Straight-backed chair
Sticky mat
Blocks (2)
Blanket (optional)
Strap (optional)

Difficulty: Any level can try this set of poses.

Set up your mat and chair so there is room for your legs on either side when you turn in your chair. Have your blocks handy.

1. Warrior I:

    a. Turn to the left and sit sideways on the edge of your chair. Place your left foot on the floor in front of you, knee bent at a right angle.

    b. Set a block on either side of your left foot.

    c. Kick your right foot back behind you, toes

on the floor. Alternatively, you can drop your right knee straight down from your hips to rest on the mat or a folded blanket.

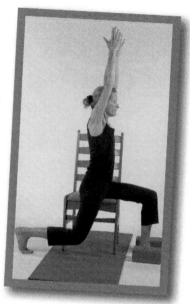

d. Allow an inhale to expand your belly, ribs, chest. Reach up with both arms, elbows straight, palms facing each other.

Seated Warrior I

2. Forward bend: Exhale, hinging at the hips, and place your hands on the blocks. Inhale up and return to center. Turn to the right and repeat Steps 1 and 2. Return to center.

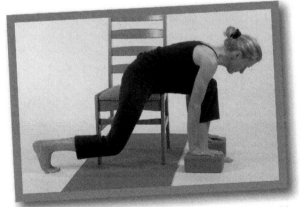

Forward bend

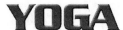
3. Take a resting breath. Notice if you sense any changes in your arms and legs.

4. Warrior II: Step your legs wide, left leg bent at a right angle at the knee, right leg straight, foot flexed and heel on the floor. Pressing down into the left foot and out through the right heel, lengthen through the crown of your head. On an inhale, raise your arms to a T position, your left arm parallel to your left knee. Relax your shoulders as you reach out through your fingertips. Gaze out over your left fingers.

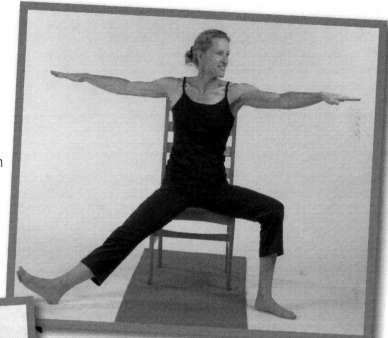

Seated Warrior II

5. Wide angle: Drop your left elbow to your left knee. On an inhale, sweep your right fingertips up, exhaling them over toward the left. Try to keep your elbow straight but not locked and your arm in line with your ear. If your neck feels comfortable, look up at your raised hand. Inhale back to center.

6. Repeat Steps 4 and 5 on the other side.

Wide-angle stretch

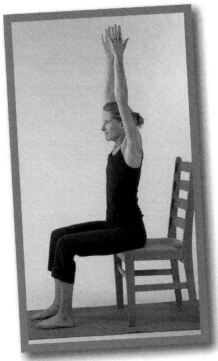

Seated Warrior III

7. Return to center and notice any sensations in your arms.

8. Warrior III: From seated mountain, inhale and raise both arms up, reaching through your fingertips and the crown of your head. Exhale and hinge forward at the hips with a straight back as you lower your upper body and extended arms toward being parallel with the floor. Note that this is an upper back strengthener. If you feel any pain in your lower back, come out of the pose and take a resting breath.

9. Yoga mudra: From Warrior III, inhale and reach your arms behind your back, interlacing your fingertips. On an exhale, point your knuckles back and up toward the ceiling. Inhale. Exhale your palms to your knees, inhaling back to upright.

- If your hands don't reach each other, feel free to use a strap. Clasp the

Yoga mudra

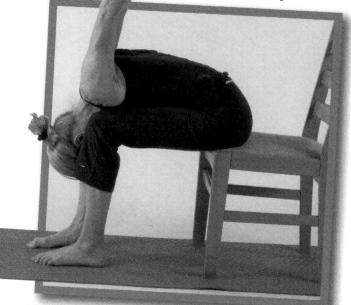

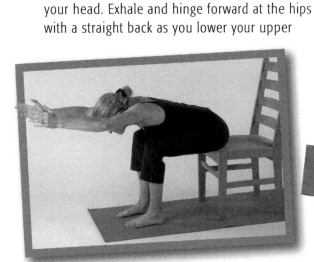

strap in each hand behind your back and point your hands back and up. Relax your arms and release the strap. Exhale your palms to your knees and inhale back to upright.

10. Bicycle legs: This is an abdominal strengthener. Place your hands behind your sitting bones on the back of the chair. Find your balance as you lift both legs, slowly pedaling an imaginary bicycle. Alternatively, keep one foot on the floor as you lift the other leg toward you, then away, before switching feet.

11. Take a resting breath and prepare for the Relaxation that follows.

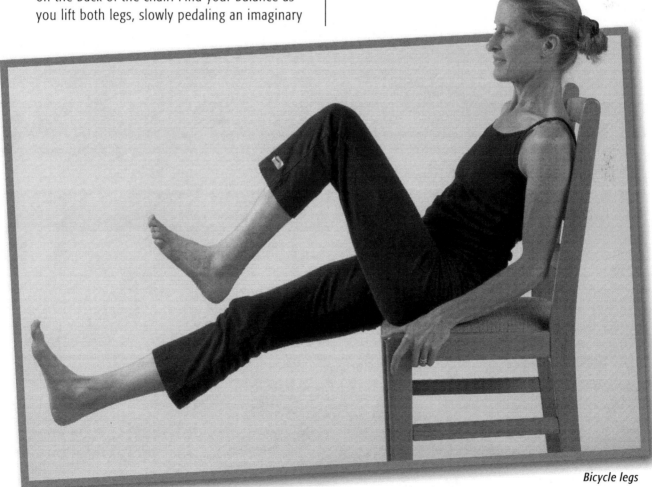

Bicycle legs

STRENGTH POSES

Standing Warrior Flow with Tree

Need: Two straight-backed chairs
Sticky mat

Difficulty: This can be a challenging and energizing flow. If you have balance or overheating concerns or are new to stretching and strengthening, try the seated variation first.

Place one chair at the end of the mat, all four legs on the mat, with the back facing you. Have the other chair handy.

1. Warrior I: Stand in mountain pose and place your hands on the chair back for support.

   a. Step your right foot back, knee straight but not locked, and press down through the heel.

   b. Bend your front knee, making sure it is lined up above your ankle, not beyond it.

   c. With equal weight pressing down though the front and back legs, raise one or both arms, elbows straight and palms facing each other. If it is comfortable for you, look up at your hands.

   d. Alternatively, keep both hands on the chair back for support and look forward or slightly up.

   e. Step back into mountain pose and switch legs, stepping your left foot back to repeat on the other side.

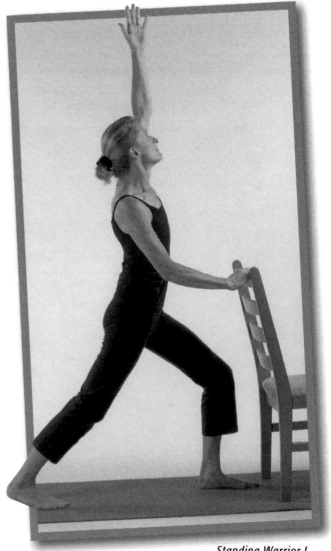

Standing Warrior I

2. Warrior II: Stand in mountain pose and place your hands on the chair back for support.

   a. Step your right food back and pivot, turning sideways to the chair.

   b. Place your left foot so it is pointing at the chair. Position your right foot so the outside is parallel to the back short end of the mat.

   c. Bend your left leg, making sure your knee is lined up above your ankle, not beyond it. Your right leg remains straight. If you can, press into the ball of the front foot and the outer edge of the back foot.

   d. With an inhale, raise your arms to a T position, your left arm parallel with your left thigh.

   e. Turn your gaze to look out over your left fingertips.

3. Wide angle: Drop your left hand to the chair for support. Inhale and raise your right arm up, exhaling it overhead. Inhale back to center and step your feet together into mountain pose. Take a resting breath.

4. Repeat Steps 2 and 3 on the other side, with your right foot pointing at the chair.

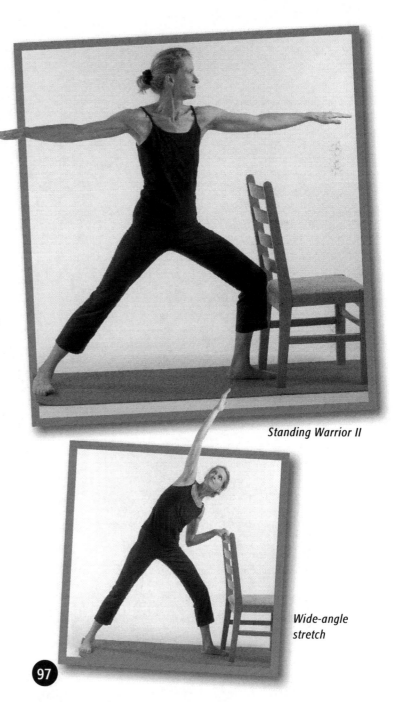

Standing Warrior II

Wide-angle stretch

The next poses are for helping and increasing balance.

5. Warrior III: Face the back of the chair.

   a. From mountain pose, place your hands on the chair back and shift your weight to one leg.

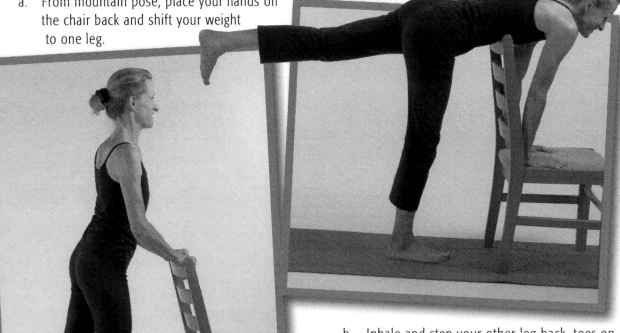

   b. Inhale and step your other leg back, toes on the mat.

   c. Exhale as you hinge forward at the hips, raising your back leg as your torso lowers. Reposition your hands on the chair as needed for support.

   d. Inhale back to mountain pose.

6. Repeat Step 5, with your weight to the other leg.

Standing Warrior III  98

7. Position the second chair opposite the first with enough room between them for you to stand between with outstretched arms. You should be able to touch the back of the chair with your fingertips for support.

8. Opposite hand to knee: Stand in mountain pose with a chair on either side of you. Raise your left knee and tap it with your right hand. Step the left foot down and raise your right knee and tap it with your left hand. Alternate between the two for four more rounds. Reach out to either chair as needed for support.

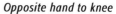

Opposite hand to knee

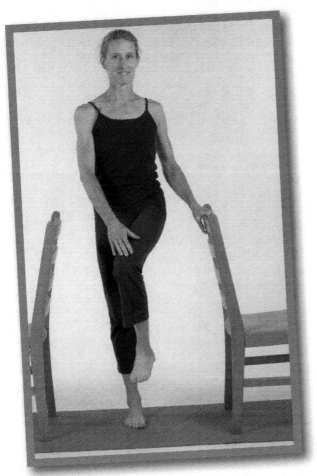

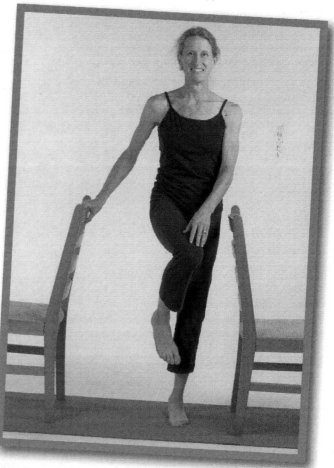

9. Turn one chair so the seat is facing forward. You may remove the second chair or keep it in place for added support.

10. Tree: Stand in mountain pose directly beside the chair.

   a. Shift your weight to the leg further from the chair.

   b. Using your hand on the chair back for support, place the leg nearest the chair on the seat, knee bent and at a right angle to your body. This stretches the inner thigh muscles.

   c. With your weight mostly on the straight leg, press down, rooting through your foot, and extend up through the crown of your head and out the bent knee, like the tree trunk, strong yet flexible.

   d. If it feels comfortable, inhale as you raise your hands overhead, fingers interlaced, index fingers pointing up.

   e. If you can, balance in tree for thirty seconds before returning to mountain pose.

   f. Take a resting breath and move to the other side of the chair for tree pose on the other leg.

11. Shake out your limbs. Remove the chair from the mat and prepare for Relaxation.

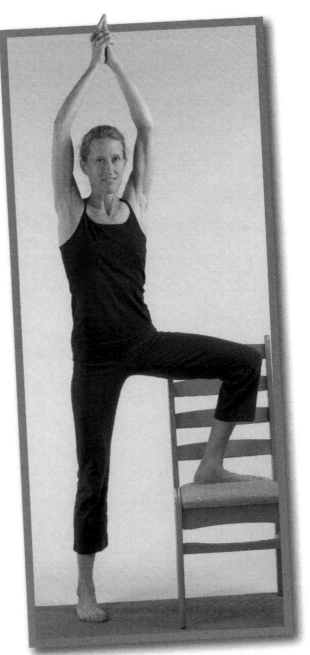

Tree

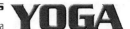
RELAXATION: GUIDED IMAGERY

Lie in a comfortable position, cushioned and supported under your head and neck and warmed by blankets. Place a bolster under your knees to relieve any strain in the lower back. Try an eye pillow (remove glasses or contact lenses first) if the room is bright.

Let yourself settle onto the mat. Feel the floor support the back of your head, shoulders, back, hips and sacrum, thighs, calves. Let them all be still, releasing into the mat, the floor, the earth.

Breathe and feel the air fill the back of your lungs, the back ribs expanding and contracting.

Allow your awareness to go to the back of your head, neck, shoulder blades. Breathe into any tension in your upper back, down the spine to the small of your back down to the tailbone. Follow your breath down the backs of your legs, hamstrings, calves, and heels. Feel them pressed into the earth, letting go.

Notice the front of your body. Feel the air on your face. Let you brows, eyes, jaw go slack. Breathe peace into any tension in your chest and shoulders, arms and open palms, abdomen, hips, thighs, shins, toes.

Supported by the earth and open to the sky, you are in the balance between what is behind you and what is before you. Like a warrior, strong while relaxed and in balance. Rest this way for several more minutes.

As you begin to bring your awareness back into the room, into your body, wiggle your fingers and toes, wrinkle up your nose. Pull one knee into your chest and then the other. Roll to one side and rest there. Note the sensations on the back of your body, on the front. How are they similar or different? Slowly push yourself up to seated and let your eyes ease open.

May you be grounded yet free. Namaste.

ESPECIALLY BENEFICIAL

- Getting up from a chair or out of bed is difficult when there's weakness on one or both sides. The warrior poses build strength in the arms and legs, which can ease the transition from sitting to standing.

- Fatigue is a common symptom of a number of movement disorders. Practicing strength and balance poses increases our stamina and can fend off fatigue.

- Balance work helps reduce falls and improves our posture.

YOGA TO GO: APPLYING IT TO YOUR DAY

- If you can, try putting your socks on while standing. Lean on a wall or stand close to the edge of the bed for safety.

- Sit in front of a mirror. Notice if you're fully upright, shoulders even. If not, before correcting yourself, close your eyes and feel the position. Open your eyes and make any adjustments. Close your eyes again and sense any difference.

• The symptoms of stroke, Parkinson's, MS and any number of movement disorders involve loss: loss of balance, muscle control, abilities. Rebuilding strength is important, but take a few moments during the day to consider the strengths you have: strength of character, a strong sense of design, a great listener and friend, an authority on roses or birds or jet engines.

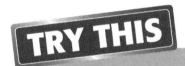

TRY THIS

TAKE FIVE

Take five minutes. Take them for yourself. Take and sit with those five minutes each day in a favorite spot. Maybe include a favorite pillow. Sit together with those five minutes as you would a dear friend, quiet together because you need no words. Sit with each other, indulging in this special time daily. Those five minutes of simply breathing reset your body, refresh your mind, and restore the mind/body connection.

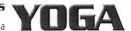
Chapter 9
FRIDAY: FLOW

'To watch us dance is to
hear our hearts speak,
– Hopi Indian saying

The first time I danced – I mean really danced with abandon – occurred seven years after my Parkinson's diagnosis.

It's not that I avoided parquet floors before then. Having two left feet – actually, only half a left foot – didn't stop me from swaying to the loud rock of college years or waddling to the chicken dance at weddings. With each step and twist, however, I was always aware that my left foot couldn't quiet keep up with the beat, that I looked awkward. And once the Parkinson's settled in, what rhythm I could muster depended on how much medication flowed into both feet.

None of that mattered at a dance for Parkinson's workshop I attended. The session required no adeptness with timing or agility or pas de deux. The class, the instructor explained, was about expression, community and motion. We marched, swayed, stomped and jigged. More importantly, we laughed – a few cried – and no one felt the least bit awkward.

ASANA PRACTICE

So much energy goes into a pose. We follow the steps, stretch an arm, straighten an elbow, align, reach and, of course, breathe. We can focus on one part of the body at a time, such as shoulders, or emphasize one action during practice, such as forward bending. Whether we're isolating areas or asanas where tension can be released or weaker areas can be strengthened or combining poses, we let the breath keep us fluid. Flow from one pose to the next. This can happen by stringing together certain poses that meld into one another. This also occurs when we stop trying so hard to *do* the pose and, instead, stay aware of our breath and let the pose happen.

With many movement disorders, motion can get jerky, awkward, stiff. Practicing yoga in a flow helps remind our muscles that they are fluid, that there is grace within. Go ahead and let those muscles dance.

Coming to Stillness

This combination of a mantra, or repeated phrase, and mudra, or hand gesture, stimulates both sides of the brain where the voice follows the breath and the finger movements flow with the voice.

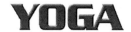
As you recite each syllable of the mantra, one fingertip on each hand touches your thumb, each time creating a circle. The mantra itself is a circle, symbolizing the cycle of life. It is *Sa Ta Na Ma* and translates as Beginning, Life, Death, and Rebirth. Like the round form the fingers and thumb make, the pattern of repetition starts where it ends.

The finger motion is

    Sa – index finger to thumb

    Ta – middle finger to thumb

    Na – ring finger to thumb

    Ma – pinkie finger to thumb

Begin in seated mountain pose with your eyes closed. Rest your hands on your lap, palms up, index finger and thumb tips touching on each hand. Take a deep breath in. On an exhale, recite the mantra as your fingers flow with each syllable of it, reciting the mantra ten times as follows:

    Two times aloud

    Two times in a whisper

    Two times silently

    Two times in whisper

    Two times aloud

When the cycle is complete, sit for a few moments, letting your breath settle back into its regular pattern.

Notice any sensations in your fingertips, any vibration in your chest. Gently open your eyes and move to the warm-ups.

Warm-ups

Please refer to Chapter 3 for the warm-up exercises to do before practicing the following flow.

Poses

This flow ends where it begins, continuing the circle. Once the steps become familiar, try repeating the flow one or more times, keeping your movements fluid. Consider playing soft music with a beat that is just right for your movement, the same piece or pieces each time, while flowing through these poses. The rhythm of the music can help cue some of the movements.

CIRCLE OF POSES

Seated Circular Flow

                Need: Straight-backed chair
                        Sticky mat

Difficulty: Any level can try this flow.

Sit in mountain pose at the edge of your chair seat.

1. **Upward salute:** Inhale as you raise both arms to the sky, palms facing upward. If it feels comfortable and you feel stable, have a look up at your hands. Turn your palms to face out and exhale your arms down.

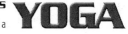
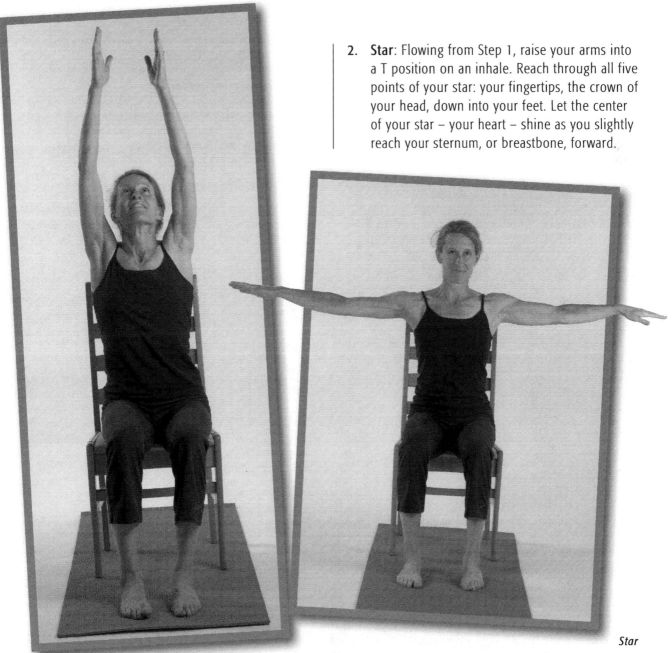

2. **Star**: Flowing from Step 1, raise your arms into a T position on an inhale. Reach through all five points of your star: your fingertips, the crown of your head, down into your feet. Let the center of your star – your heart – shine as you slightly reach your sternum, or breastbone, forward.

Seated circular flow: upward salute

Star

3. **Stargazer**: Keeping your arms straight, inhale while you raise your right fingertips to the sky, your left to the ground.

Look up at your right fingertips. Exhale back to star and inhale your left fingertips to the sky.

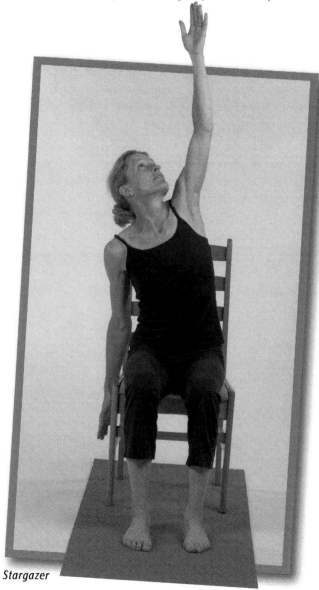

Stargazer

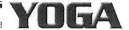
4. **Twist**: Inhale back to star. Bend your elbows and place your fingertips on your shoulders. Following your breath, inhale center and exhale and twist to one side; inhale center, exhale and twist to the other side. Repeat three times, ending on a twist to the right.

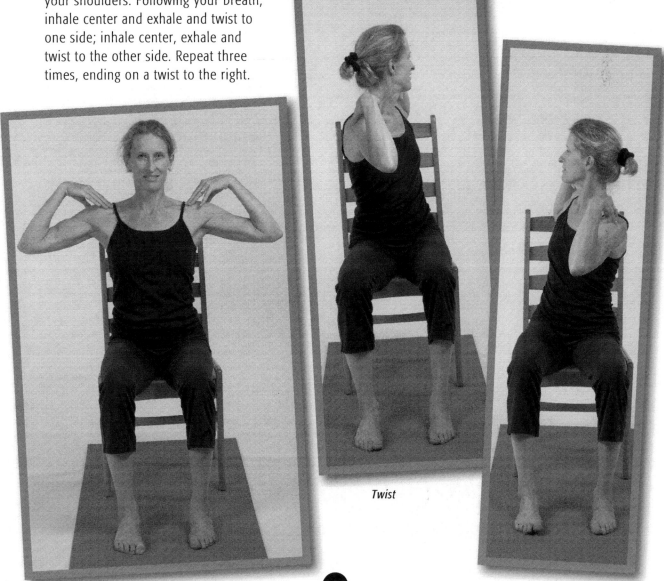

Twist

5. **Wide-angle stretch**: Straighten your right arm and gaze out over your right fingertips. Inhale and raise your right arm straight overhead. Exhale as you bend your upper body, reaching your fingers toward your left knee. On an inhale, straighten, and repeat the twist in Step 4 two more times, ending on the left. Repeat the wide-angle stretch for the left arm.

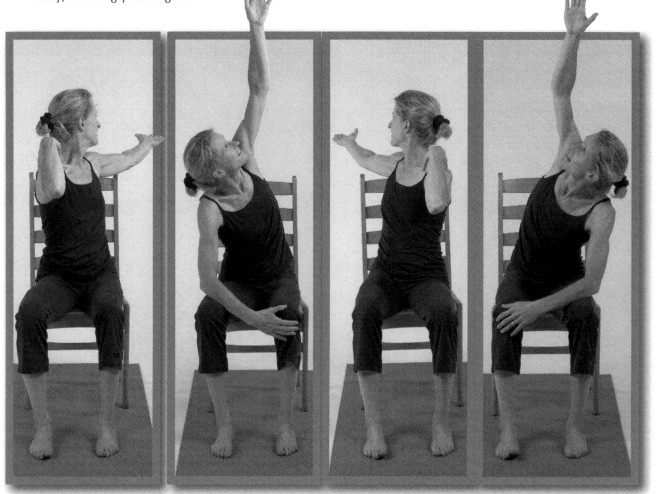

Wide-angle stretch

6. **Clasped-hands shoulder release**: Flowing from Step 5, straighten back to center, raising both arms overhead on an inhale, clasping your fingers together and turning palms up. Reach through your hands and the crown of your head, keeping your shoulders relaxed. Exhale your arms in front of you, fingers still clasped but palms turned in to face you. Let your upper back round and drop your chin slightly, opening up the shoulder blades. Inhale as you release your clasp and bring your hands behind your back, once again clasping your fingers, palms facing your back. Exhale your elbows straight as you raise your sternum and gaze slightly.

- If your hands don't reach behind your back, use a strap. Clasp the strap behind your back where it is comfortable for your hands.

7. Release and inhale back to seated mountain pose.

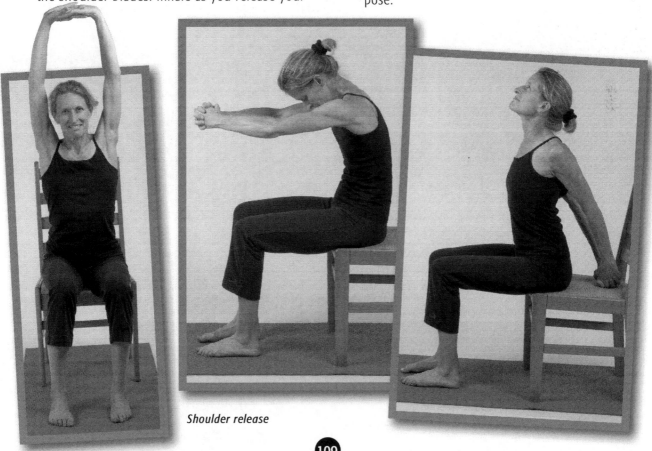

Shoulder release

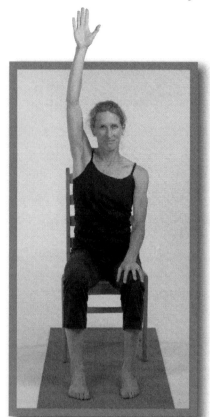
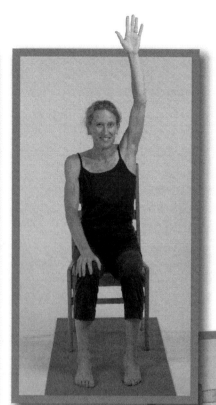
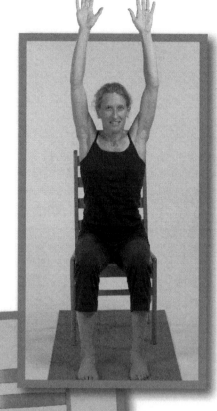

Raised arms

8. **Arms up**: Release your hands to your knees. Inhale and sweep your right hand overhead, exhaling your hand back to your knee. Inhale and sweep your left hand overhead, exhaling back to your knee. Inhale and sweep both hands overhead, exhaling into a forward bend, hinging from the hips with a straight back.

9. **Upward salute**: Inhale up, raising your arms to the sky, palms facing upward.

10. Exhale arms down, back to seated mountain, and take a resting breath before preparing for the Relaxation that follows.

RELAXATION: GUIDED IMAGERY

As you adjust to lying on your mat, feel the floor beneath you, solid. Let your whole body – your head, shoulders, back, legs – be fully supported and cushioned by blankets or a bolster. Inhale deeply through your nose, pause, and exhale it all out through your mouth.

Close your eyes and let them relax. Allow your jaw to soften, your forehead to be smooth. Imagine a mountain stream. Picture the stream at its beginning, at a waterfall high up in the rocks. Clean, clear water. Listen as it rushes between the rocks, splashing into a pool below. Watch as a droplet springs from the waterfall and dances and swirls in the stream that flows past roots and pebbles, through the countryside into a lake at the base of the mountain. On a warm day, the drop evaporates before it condenses again in a cloud that will send it back to the waterfall. Now watch as a droplet from the waterfall lands on the crown of your head. It flows through you, dancing and swirling into any space that needs fluidity. Let it wash into your lower back or across your knees, gliding in, clean and clear. Watch as the droplet reenters the stream that flows to the lake. Rest for a few more minutes knowing that the cycle will continue, that you are fluid.

As you begin to bring your awareness back to the room, take several deep breaths. Wiggle your fingers and toes, wrinkle up your nose. Pull one knee up to your chest and then the other. Give yourself a hug and rock slightly from side to side. Before you sit up and open your eyes, notice if any part of you feels lighter, freer, more fluid.

May peace flow like a river within you. Namaste.

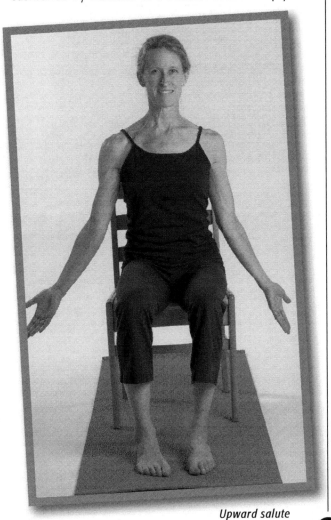

Upward salute

ESPECIALLY BENEFICIAL

- Some movement disorders affect the strength of our voices. Like singing, chanting mantras increases our lung capacity and diaphragm control, both of which contribute to strong vocal projection.

- Rigidity and involuntary contractions can soften with repetitive flowing movements.

- Connecting rhythmic movements to the regular beat of music can help with motor block. Moving to the familiar beat of a song can help set us in motion when we're feeling "stuck."

YOGA TO GO: APPLYING IT TO YOUR DAY

- Ask your doctor if dancing is right for you.

- Drink a glass of water. Taste it. Feel it on your tongue and as it goes down your throat.

- Bring your attention to your breath as you listen to water falling – raindrops, a shower, a melting icicle. Notice the pattern, the rhythm of the water. Notice the pattern, the rhythm of your breath.

- If you experience dyskinesia, try listening to a favorite song or two and allowing the dyskinetic motion to happen in rhythm with the music.

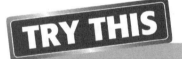

GREEN RICE

Studies suggest that green tea's antioxidants may be helpful to people with Parkinson's because they protect dopamine neurons. Besides a cup or two in the morning, try leftover green tea in soups or in lieu of water when cooking grains (green tea with jasmine makes for flavorful rice).

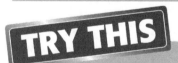

RHYTHM ON THE GO

Consider carrying a music player wherever you go. When you're "off," moving particularly slowly or get "stuck," turn to the beat for help. Sort your playlists by the pace. Choose a quick beat when you need to rush through the airport. When there's no hurry, you can still benefit from the cues that a more moderate rhythm can provide.

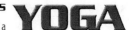
Chapter 10
SATURDAY: RESTORE

'Renew thyself completely each day:
do it again, again, and forever again,
– Chinese inscription cited by Thoreau in *Walden*

Before class begins, the studio is quiet as people ease into stretches or simply sit on their chairs, absorbed in the moment.

Enter: Joe. A new student with a round, boyish face and an impish grin, he is talking to anyone and everyone. Laughing and chattering, he takes a seat. Sentences continue to crash into one another well into the warm-ups. His stroke has clearly not affected his speech.

We move through neck and shoulder rolls. Small pockets of stillness settle between his words. As we gently work through seated poses, there are longer pauses. I watch his shoulders drop, his fingers unfurl as he relaxes in the chair.

When it is time for an ending restorative pose, he lies back on the mat, a blanket rolled up under his knees, another folded for a pillow, a lighter one draped across him. He does not speak. He simply breathes.

The restorative power of a fully supported pose grounded him, released him from the nervousness that can throw any of us off balance and cause us to prattle on too much or too fast. He later said he slept quite well that night. Now that's something to talk about.

ASANA PRACTICE

Restorative poses differ from regular asanas. Rather than actively reaching and stretching, restorative poses passively allow opening to occur. The body rests in any of a number of positions propped by blankets, bolsters, rolled-up towels, pillows, weighted bags. Gravity and the deepening breath allow for release. Grounded by the earth solid beneath us, restoratives help renew the smallest cells and bring light to the darkest mood. No need to wait until the end of the week to enjoy these poses.

Coming to Stillness

Before finding a comfortable seated position, choose one of the following poses and set up your props for it. That way, you can move smoothly from a relaxed position into the few warm-ups and on to the restorative pose. These asanas are somewhat labor-intensive to set up, with lots of folding and positioning of props. But, they're well worth the effort once you've settled into the supported pose.

Once you've arranged your blankets and blocks, find a comfortable, straight-backed position on a cushion, on the mat or on a chair, with your palms resting on your knees or with your hands on a pillow in your lap. If you're on a chair, position your hips at the rear of the chair seat so that your spine can rest on the back of the chair. If you're on a cushion or the mat, consider sitting so that your back is against a wall for added support.

Gently lengthen your spine by reaching up through the crown of your head while pressing down through your sitting bones.

Allow your eyes to close. Soften the muscles in your face: your brow, your jaw. Feel your body supported from below and from behind. Notice if you can feel your feet in contact with the floor, your sitting bones against the cushion or mat. Allow yourself to sink into the support, settling down and back.

Inhale deeply and pause your breath to the count of two. Let your exhale be an audible *ahh*. Inhale and exhale this way two more times.

Warm-ups

Working through a few warm-ups before a restorative pose opens up the spine and can help align joints. This provides for a deeper relaxation during the restorative pose. Rather than following the full routine of warm-ups, move through 7, 8, and 9 from Set A and 2 and 4 from Set B (please refer to Chapter 3 for the warm-up exercises).

Poses

Four poses are listed here. Each has a different restorative benefit. Choose the one that best fits your needs at the moment. The first is a calming pose, the second refreshes, and the third pose is nurturing.

SUPPORTED BASIC RELAXATION

Floor Variation
(Or, couch or bed variation)

> *Need: Bolsters or sofa cushions*
> *Blankets and towels (up to 5)*
> *Sandbag or bag of rice (optional)*
> *Eye pillow (optional)*
> *Timer (optional)*

Difficulty: Anyone can try all four of these poses.

In this first position, bolsters and blankets support your body as you lie on your back. This is an overall calming pose that can help slow your heart rate and quiet the central nervous system.

The floor's solidity provides better support for this pose, but if getting down onto the floor is difficult, this position can be done on a couch or in bed.

Set up the resting – or what I like to refer to as *nesting* – space by spreading a blanket, folded in two lengthwise, on the floor for cushioning. Place small towels or washcloths folded once on either side of

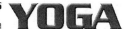
the blanket, about midway down. These will support your wrists.

If your legs need added support, have two sandbags or sacks of rice ready near the foot of your blanket. These can be placed at the outside of your legs, along the knees and shins, to keep your legs from rolling out too much.

Have a bolster or sofa cushion handy to place under your knees.

Fold another blanket or towel for your head and neck. Be sure that the folds provide enough support so that your chin points directly toward the ceiling, not tilting back or tucked forward. If you'd like, have an eye pillow or washcloth folded lengthwise handy for lightly covering your eyes (remove glasses or contacts first).

You may want to set a timer. If you do, try to use one that has a peaceful sound rather than a jarring one so that you're not jolted out of your relaxed state.

Finally, have another blanket ready for covering up against cold. It is important not to get chilled because it will become too difficult to relax. Also, with Parkinson's and with MS, body temperature regulation gets off kilter and once the body gets cold, it can take some time to get warm again.

Once the props are in place, consider using the bolster to sit on for Coming to Stillness so that it is a smooth transition to this restorative pose.

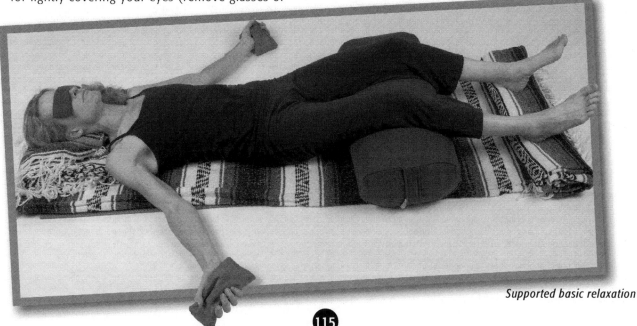

Supported basic relaxation

1. After the three rounds of breath in Coming to Stillness, slide off the bolster down to the blanket. Arrange the bolster under your knees and the sandbags or sacks of rice, if you're using them, beside your legs.

2. Place your wrist supports in position so that you can reach them once you've reclined.

3. Use a blanket to cover yourself to keep warm if the room is at all cool.

4. Lie back and rest your head on the folded towel or blanket and place the eye pillow or folded washcloth over your eyes to block the light. Rest your wrists on the small folded towels or washcloths.

5. Breathe. Inhale and pause as you did in Coming to Stillness. Exhale with an audible *ahh*. Let your entire body – bones, tissue, organs – all settle into the supports. Smile. Feel that smile travel to your bones, tissue, organs.

6. Breathe your normal breath and relax in this pose for at least fifteen minutes. Twenty would be okay, too. So would thirty.

7. To ease out of the pose, keep your eyes closed as you wiggle your fingers and toes. Remove the eye pillow and scrunch up your nose.

8. Take a deep breath in and out. Pull one knee to your chest. Push the bolster away slightly with your other leg before pulling that knee to your chest, hugging both knees in. Roll to one side and rest there for a moment.

9. Pressing your hands into the floor, push yourself up and sit for a moment. Notice your breath and the sounds around you. Bring your awareness to your body, to the ease that has settled in, even a little. When you're ready, open your eyes and rejoin the world.

INVERTED RESTORATIVE POSE

Elevated Legs

> *Need: Blankets (2)*
> *Chair or sofa or bed*
> *Sandbag or sack of rice (optional)*
> *Eye pillow (optional), Timer (optional)*

In elevated legs pose, the feet are positioned higher than the heart, inverting blood flow. This can reduce swelling in the ankles and help with restless, involuntary movements in the leg muscles. It can be used to refresh after overdoing. Please note: anyone with glaucoma or high blood pressure should check with a doctor before practicing this pose. Also, if you have a head cold or sinus infection, avoid this pose until you've recovered.

Set up for this pose by spreading a blanket, folded in two lengthwise, on the floor for cushioning. Place a straight-backed chair on one end of the blanket, or spread the blanket perpendicular to the edge of a sofa or bed.

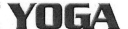
Place one small towel or washcloth, folded once, on either side of the blanket, about a foot from the chair, sofa, or bed. These will support your wrists. Have another blanket handy if needed to cover up to stay warm. If you're using a timer, have that handy as well.

Fold another blanket or towel for your head and neck. Be sure that the folds provide enough support so that your chin points directly toward the ceiling, not tilting back or tucked forward. If you'd like, have an eye pillow or washcloth folded lengthwise handy for lightly covering your eyes (remove glasses or contacts first).

Once the props are in place, consider using the chair (or sofa or bed) to sit on for Coming to Stillness so that it is a smooth transition to this restorative pose.

1. After the three rounds of breath in Coming to Stillness, gently come off the chair and lie down on the blanket on your back, facing the chair. Swing your legs up onto the seat of the chair, knees bent and calves comfortably supported.

2. If you're using a sandbag, place it across your shins. This helps keep your legs stable, allowing your hips and thighs to completely let go of doing any of the work keeping your legs in place.

3. Adjust the blanket under your head and neck for comfort and chin alignment.

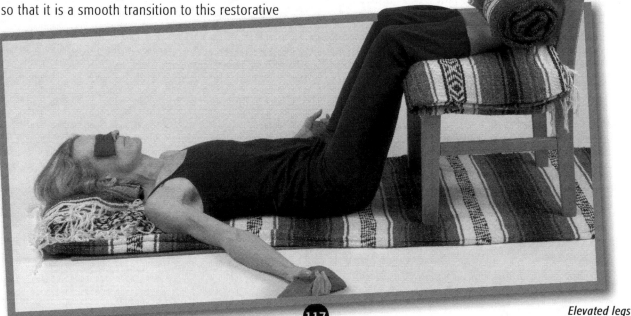

Elevated legs

4. Place your wrist supports in position so that you can reach them once you've reclined.

5. Use a blanket to cover yourself to keep warm if the room is at all cool.

6. Lie back and rest your head on the folded towel or blanket and place the eye pillow or folded washcloth over your eyes to block the light. Rest your wrists on the small folded towels or washcloths.

7. Breathe. Inhale and pause as you did in Coming to Stillness. Exhale with an audible *ahh*. Let your entire body – bones, tissue, organs – all settle into the supports. Smile. Feel that smile travel to your bones, tissue, organs.

8. Breathe your normal breath and relax in this pose for ten to fifteen minutes. Twenty would be okay, too. Come out of the pose if your toes begin to tingle from lack of blood.

9. To ease out of the pose, keep your eyes closed and wiggle your fingers and toes. Remove the eye pillow and scrunch up your nose.

10. Take a deep breath in and out. Wriggle your legs out from under the sandbag if you're using one. Pull one knee to your chest and then the other, hugging both knees in. Roll to one side and rest there for a moment.

11. Pressing your hands into the floor, push yourself up and sit for a moment. Give your circulation a chance to readjust. Notice your breath. Bring your awareness to your body, to any spark of new energy. With a smile, open your eyes and continue living your day.

SEATED RESTORATIVE POSE

Child's Pose in a Chair

Need: Two straight-backed chairs
Sticky mat, Bolster or sofa cushion
Block or book(s), Blankets or towels

This restorative pose is akin to a grown-up's version of a Time Out. It can reset your mood and bring you back into balance. It also opens up the back muscles while cradling the heart and mind.

To set up for this pose, place two chairs eight to ten inches apart, seats facing each other. Turn one chair slightly so a corner of the seat is facing the other chair. Both chairs should have all four legs on the mat to prevent slippage.

Place a block or books on the back of the seat of the chair that is not turned. Place the bolster or sofa cushion beside the chairs.

Fold the blanket or towel to fit the length of the bolster. If it is a long blanket, fold the end several times to form a pillow for supporting your head on the bolster. If the blanket is not long enough, fold a towel for your head to rest on.

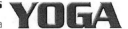

Have an extra two blankets or blocks handy if your feet do not rest comfortably on the floor when seated in the chair. Have your timer within reach, if you are using one.

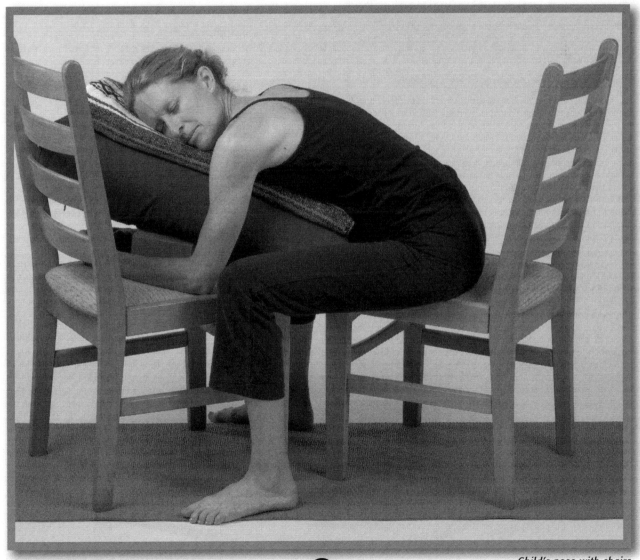

Child's pose with chairs

For a smooth transition to this restorative pose, consider using the chair that is turned to sit on for Coming to Stillness. Sit so that one of your legs is on each side of the corner of the seat that points to the other chair.

1. After the three rounds of breath in Coming to Stillness, reach for the bolster. Place one end on the corner of the chair you're sitting on and the other end on the block or books on the other chair.

2. Position the blanket and or towels on the bolster for your head support.

3. Check the position of your legs. Your knees and ankles should each be at right angles. If your legs are short, place a block or blanket or pillow under your feet until you get the correct angle of ankle and knee.

4. Bend forward to rest your belly and chest on the bolster, turning your head to rest on a cheek, and looping your arms under the bolster between the block and where it is resting on the seat of the chair. Let your shoulders droop and relax. Notice if there is any discomfort and rearrange props as needed.

5. Breathe. Inhale and pause as you did in Coming to Stillness. Exhale with an audible *ahh*. Let your entire body – bones, tissue, organs – all settle onto the supports. Close your eyes and let everything go quiet, all the chatter in your mind

fall silent. Feel that stillness travel to your bones, tissue, organs.

6. Breathe your normal breath and relax in this pose for ten to fifteen minutes. Halfway through, turn your head to rest on the other cheek.

7. To ease out of the pose, keep your eyes closed and wiggle your fingers and toes. Scrunch up your nose.

8. Take a deep breath in and out. Stretch your arms out in front of you or to the sides.

9. Pressing your hands into the bolster, push yourself up and sit for a moment. Notice your first thought. Smile at it. Bring your awareness to your body, to any place that has settled into ease. Your Time Out is over. Open your eyes and enjoy your time back in your day.

RECLINING RESTORATIVE POSE

Need: Bolster or sofa cushion
Blocks or books (4-6)
Blankets (2-3)
Eye pillows

This variation on the reclined bound-angle pose is heavily supported. Some of my students refer to this as the lounge chair pose. Blankets, cushions and blocks encourage the head, back, hips, knees to let go, to create an openness in areas that are particularly tight or contracted from dystonia.

The eye pillows are for the palms of the hands to help release gripping or tremors. The extra blocks support the arms to relieve any strain in the shoulders (shoulder pain is a common secondary symptom of Parkinson's and the shoulders can be difficult to relax if affected by a stroke).

1. Begin by arranging the props. Set the bolster lengthwise on the mat. Place a cushion or folded blanket at the head of the bolster. Set two blocks in their flattest position short-end-to-short-end on either side of the mat. The other two are at the foot of the mat awaiting positioning. Set an eye pillow on each set of blocks along the sides of the mat and bolster.

2. Ease into the pose. First. sit on the mat with the back of your hips abutting the short end of the bolster. Next, with the soles of the feet touching, bring the two blocks from the foot of the mat to beneath each thigh just above the bent knee. The block can be positioned to whatever height is needed to fully support the legs. There should be no strain, no active holding in the inner thigh muscles.

3. From here, lie back slowly, easing the spine onto the bolster. It is important that the bolster doesn't move or slide up the mat as the body eases on to it. If possible, have another person

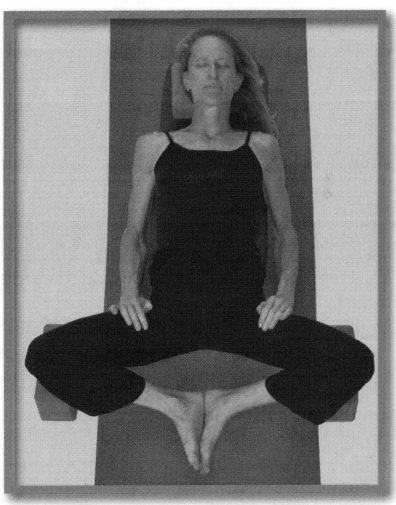

Reclining restorative pose

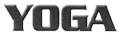
hold the bolster in place during this step. Or, try arranging the top end of the bolster against the wall before this step.

4. Allow your head to be supported by the cushion or blanket so that the neck is neutral, not overextending but also not with the chin tucked.

5. Take hold of an eye pillow in each hand. Rest the forearms and wrists on the sets of two blocks. Allow the palms to be face up and soften the grip on the eye pillows. Let them merely rest on the palms.

6. Breathe and allow for the softening that gravity provides. Remain in this pose as long as you are comfortable but try not to exceed fifteen minutes.

7. To come out of this pose, release the eye pillows. Remove the blocks from under the thighs. Move one set of arm blocks aside and roll off the bolster to that side. Curl into a fetal position for several breaths before moving into an upright, seated position. And before rising, allow a few cycles of breath to notice the openings, to drink them in.

ESPECIALLY BENEFICIAL

- Relaxation is a key component of boosting the immune system and allowing for healing. Living with a movement disorder does not grant us a Get Out of Jail Free card for other illnesses or diseases. We still catch colds. Through relaxation techniques, such as regularly practicing restorative poses, you help your body stay strong.

- A fully relaxed mind and body will aid in both falling asleep and staying asleep for longer periods. This is particularly helpful for the insomnia often attached to Parkinson's or from side effects of movement disorder medications.

- Releasing tension throughout the body can ease tremor and involuntary muscle contractions.

- The rejuvenation that can come with the elevated legs pose can be a welcome bit of energy when fatigued.

- Restfulness in the face of stress is just plain good for ourselves and everyone around us.

YOGA TO GO: APPLYING IT TO YOUR DAY

- If you drive, de-stress your car time. Drive at the speed limit. On the highway, let other cars pass with the same detachment as if leaves were blowing by. Give yourself a few minutes extra to enjoy the ride.

- Create a morning ritual that is calming. Before getting out of bed, close your eyes and listen to your breathing. How quiet can you make it?

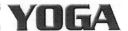
Follow the sound inside. Notice any sensations in your body – cool air on your skin, an ache. Without judgment, breathe into those spaces. Smile.

• Take a moment in the beginning of your day to pause. Choose a place to sit for a couple of minutes – in your kitchen, outside in the yard, on a step – and close your eyes. When you open them, make note of the first color you see. Think of something that color that is soothing. Notice how many times you see that color during the day.

• Breathe. Notice when your breath is short or shallow. Treat yourself to a deep inhale and equally or longer deep exhale, at the grocery store, folding laundry, while working on the computer.

• Smile and laugh. Often.

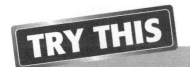

TAKE CARE

Get a pedicure. Or at least soak your feet, massage them, rub lotion into the rough spots. With movement disorders, we sometimes forget about our feet. There are so many muscles and joints throughout the body to orchestrate simply to walk or climb a flight of stairs that our feet get left out in the cold. Or, always hidden away in socks. In yoga, we're grounded by our feet, even in many seated positions. Although the sensations aren't what they once were, there is still blood flowing into our toes, a set of nerves on our soles, a pulse at our ankles. Let energy flow between you and the ground. Expose your toes. Go barefoot. Feel the earth under your feet.

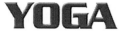
Chapter 11
MEDITATION AND MORE

'Yoga is a light, which once lit, will never dim. The better your practice, the brighter the flame,
– B. K. S. Iyengar

Mornings are my favored time to practice yoga. I try to schedule meetings for afternoons to keep the beginning of the day open. The week's calendar doesn't always work out that way. Still, I try to get a few minutes on the mat before having to dash off.

One morning, while driving to an appointment half an hour away, my mind wandered in and out of a variety of musings. Items on my to-do list, wondering what I'd eat for lunch, reactions to the news on the radio all bounced across my brain. After twenty minutes, I pulled up behind a row of cars at a stop light. My shoulders felt as though they'd tensed up to my ears. My fingers squeezed the steering wheel. I glanced out at the bumper sticker of the car in front of me. It read: Don't Believe Everything You Think.

I laughed. I felt the tension ease. I wanted to thank the driver for bringing me back to the moment. While traveling to my appointment, my mind was anywhere but there in the car seat with my body.

Meditation practice on the mat – or on a chair or lying down – is a tool to help keep us in the moment throughout our daily activities. Thoughts happen.

Meditation teaches us to step back and watch them happen and recognize we are more than our to-do lists.

BEGINNING YOUR PRACTICE

Meditation still comes as a challenge to me. But one early morning when I awoke to a quiet house, I swung my legs over the side of the bed, wrapped myself in a quilt, and followed my breath in and out. When the song lyric that had plagued me for two days started repeating itself, I focused on my breath. Thoughts swam in. *Don't forget to call about the gutters. Bring a salad to Beth's tonight.* I didn't wave them away or get annoyed. Instead, I recognized them as thoughts and brought myself back to the air moving in and out with each breath. A tremor crept into my thumb, settled in my wrist. I breathed into it.

When I opened my eyes, I stretched my arms out and glanced at the clock. Ten minutes had gone by. I'd done it; I'd *meditated.* Had I experienced an awakening? No. Though I did wonder about what my thoughts said about me and my state of being. *Gutters? Salad?*

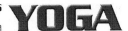
But that's one of the points about meditation. We are not our thoughts—thankfully, or I'd be pretty dull given what popped into my head. Past events or conversations replay in our minds. Or, if you're more of a planner, future events or conversations preview in your head. In either case, we really have no control. How many times have I wished something would stay as it was, or expected an outcome and was disappointed when it didn't happen as I'd hoped? Coming back to the breath brings us back to the present moment, because the present moment is all that we truly have.

In meditation, we step back into a witness role and watch those thoughts of past and future, let them come and go without getting caught up in them. Simply notice them and gently return awareness to the breath.

When and Where

When we think of yoga we typically envision moving our bodies into various poses. The original yogis of the past, however, meditated. They developed asana practice years later to stretch before or between sittings so they could meditate for longer periods. Meditation came first.

Deciding where to add a meditation period – before or after or even at a separate time from your asana practice – is a personal choice. Early morning has the advantage that it may be the quietest time with least distractions. On the other hand, my muscles are eager to go with the first light of day and

I find it easier to sit after I've moved around for an hour or so.

The length of time and number of times a day or per week that you meditate is different for each of us. Starting with ten minutes a few times a week is a good beginning. Expand the length or number of days as you feel comfortable. Or, if you tend to get overly stiff from not moving, try sitting for ten minutes several times during the day rather than sitting for an hour at a time.

Props

You can sit or lie down for meditation, though, often, when I lie down I fall asleep. I find that sitting on a straight-backed chair is best for comfort, though I do sit on the edge of the bed at times. A pillow in your lap makes a good support for resting your arms. If your legs are short, use a folded blanket or firm pillow under your feet to bring your legs to a position where there are right angles at the ankles, knees, and hips. Keep another blanket handy in case you feel chilled while sitting.

The keys to staying alert are to maintain a straight spine and to be comfortable. Even with the softest pillows and the best intentions, though, the mind has a tendency to wander. Stephen Cope, a psychotherapist and senior Kripalu yoga teacher, likens sitting for meditation as tying a puppy to a post. Our puppy minds are active; they especially object and tug at their collars when we tie them up and say, Stay. But, eventually, our endless thoughts, like the puppy, will lie down and relax.

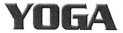
TECHNIQUES

There are numerous styles, approaches to, and venues for meditation. If you're interested in learning more, yoga studios, various churches, and continuing education courses offer classes. Group meditation guided by an instructor can be a helpful way of staying focused.

If you're distracted by someone coughing or breathing deeply, you may prefer sitting solo. There are audio CDs available that lead you through meditation steps and visualizations. Choose what works best for you. Listed here are only a few of the many meditation techniques.

In and Out

Need: A straight-backed chair or a cushion
Blanket or pillow (optional)

This technique is one that I come back to again and again for its simplicity. It uses the breath as the focal point. Once you are in a comfortable seated position, close your eyes or let the lids drift partway closed. Inhale a full, slow breath through the nose and say to yourself, "In." As you exhale through the nose, slowly and fully, say to yourself, "Out."

Thich Nhat Hanh, a Vietnamese monk, Zen master and author adds to this. After several rounds of breath, inhale a full, slow breath through the nose and say to yourself, "In. Relax." And, on the exhale, say to yourself, "Out. Smile."

To end your session, sit for another moment and notice if anything feels different: lighter or heavier, warmer or cooler. Slowly open your eyes. Smile.

Object

Need: A straight-backed chair or a cushion
Blanket or pillow (optional)

This technique uses a visual to focus on during the meditation. The object can be a candle, a vase of flowers, a postcard of a place you've been, a photo of someone you love, a seashell. Once you're in a comfortable, seated position, gaze at the object for several breaths. Next, gently close your eyes and keep the image in your mind. Continue your slow, steady breathing as you picture the object. If your mind wanders or you need a reminder of what the object's details are, open your eyes part way and glance at the object before closing your eyes again.

To end your session, sit for another moment and notice how your body feels. Mentally scan from your head to your toes. Is your jaw relaxed, your brow not furrowed? Does your back feel ready to bend and move? Are there any other sensations you notice?

Visualization

Need: A straight-backed chair or a cushion
Blanket or pillow (optional)

For this technique, you use your imagination to envision relaxation and healing. Settle into a comfortable seated position. As you breathe, focus on a particular ache or area of your body. Picture

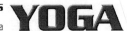
the ache or sore area as a new bud, still tightly closed. Imagine the warmth of the sun on the bud and picture it gently opening into a flower. Or, use another image of something taut that you'd like loosened, such as a gnarled fist into a smooth open palm, a butterfly emerging from a cocoon, snow melting and evaporating.

To end your session, sit for another moment with the open image in your mind – the flower in full bloom, for example. Really let yourself see it so you can recall that soft, smooth image any time during the day.

ESPECIALLY BENEFICIAL

- The visualization technique helps break up the knots that build up from involuntary muscle contractions.

- Allow your visualization to include the images of any or all of the areas in your body that have been working well, fluidly, pain-free. Take a moment to notice, even to thank them.

- As meditation practice becomes a part of your day, like brushing your teeth, you'll find you don't want to skip a session. A daily practice relaxes us in mind and body on a regular basis, keeping stress levels down.

- Your constant companion is you. Meditation lets you tap into that essence and be with it without judgment.

MEDITATION TO GO: APPLYING IT TO YOUR DAY

- The In and Out technique is available at any time of day. Try it for a few breaths at the dinner table, in the shower, at the corner store.

- There is plenty to explore to deepen your knowledge of yoga and meditation: classes, books, DVDs. These resources cover material from an in-depth study of the breath to the essence of yoga, to its history, to variations on poses and the limbs of yoga.

My fears and worries don't disappear during meditation. They still exist, but the calm that comes with a session allows me to step back, bring the fears and worries into balance. It's like rearranging the letters in an anagram, making one word or phrase from the same letters as another. The tiger is always there. But I've reordered its hold on me. It's no coincidence that *meditation* is an anagram of *no, I tamed it*.

Whatever it is that you want to tame, wherever you choose to go with yoga and meditation, breathe and enjoy your journey.

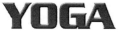
Bibliography

Cappy, P. (2006) *Yoga for All of Us: A Modified Series of Traditional Poses for Any Age and Ability.* New York, NY: St. Martin's Press.

Christensen, A. (1999) *The American Yoga Association's Easy Does It Yoga.* New York, NY: Fireside.

Cope, S. (2006) *The Wisdom of Yoga: A Seeker's Guide to Extraordinary Living.* New York, NY: Bantam.

Devi, N. (2000). *The Healing Path of Yoga: Alleviate Stress, Open Your Heart, and Enrich Your Life.* New York: Three Rivers Press.

Farhi, D. (2003) *Bringing Yoga to Life: The Everyday Practice of Enlightened Living.* New York, NY: Harper Collins.

——— (2000) *Yoga Mind, Body & Spirit: A Return to Wholeness.* New York, NY: Henry Holt and Company.

Folan, L. (2005) *Yoga Gets Better with Age.* Emmaus, PA: Rodale Press.

Goodwin V. A., et al. "The effectiveness of exercise intervention for people with Parkinson's disease: A systematic review." *Movement Disord.* 2008; 23(5):631-640.

Hackney, M. E., et al. "Effects of tango on functional mobility in Parkinson's disease: A preliminary study." *Journal of Neurological Physical Therapy*, Vol. 31, December 2007.

Hanh, T. (1991) *Peace Is Every Step: The Path of Mindfulness in Everyday Life.* New York, NY: Bantam.

Iyengar, B. K. S. (2008) *Yoga, The Path to Holistic Health.* London: D K Publishing.

Kraftsow, G. (1999) *Yoga for Wellness: Healing with the Timeless Teachings of Viniyoga*: New York, NY: Penguin Group.

Lasater, J. (2003) *30 Essential Yoga Poses: For Beginning Students and Their Teachers.* Berkeley, CA: Rodmell Press.

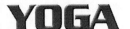
——— (1995) *Relax & Renew*: Yoga for Stressful Times. Berkeley, CA: Rodmell Press.

Le Verrier, R. Namasta: North American Studio Alliance. "Your Yoga Studio: Setting Up a User-Friendly Environment for All Abilities." 2011: http://www.namasta.com/User-Friendly-Yoga-Studio.php.

Long, R. (2006) *The Key Muscles of Hatha Yoga*. Plattsburgh, NY: BandaYoga.

McCall, T. (2007) *Yoga as Medicine: The Yogic Prescription for Health and Healing.* New York, NY: Bantam.

Oken B. S., Kishiyama S., Zajdel D., et al. "Randomized controlled trial of yoga and exercise in multiple sclerosis." *Neurology* 2004 Jun 8;62(11):2058-64.

Parkinson's Disease & Movement Disorder Society of India: Iyengar Yogashraya, Light on Yoga Research Trust. "Yoga & Parkinson's Disease." http://www.parkinsonssocietyindia.com/Yoga_Parkinson_Disease.aspx.

Sacks, O. (2007) *Musicophilia: Tales of Music and the Brain*. New York, NY: Knopf.

Schmid, A., et al. *Preliminary Evidence of Yoga on Balance and Endurance Outcomes for Veterans with Stroke* (Abstract #3157). Presented at the Annual Meeting of the American College of Sports Medicine (ACSM), June, 2011.

Searls, Y. University of Kansas. *The Therapeutic Effects of Yoga for People with Parkinson's Disease.* http://clinicaltrials.gov/ct2/show/NCT00312559.

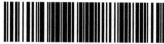

Made in the USA
San Bernardino, CA
22 September 2016